SURGICAL ANATO

SURGICAL ANATOMY OF THE ABDOMEN

Editors:

MIRCEA BEURAN

IONUȚ NEGOI

THE PUBLISHING HOUSE OF THE ROMANIAN ACADEMY
Bucharest, 2016

THE PUBLISHING HOUSE OF THE ROMANIAN ACADEMY
Calea 13 Septembrie no 13, 5ᵗʰ District
050711, Bucharest, Romania
Phone: 4021-318 81 46, 4021-318 81 06
Fax: 4021-318 24 44
E-mail: edacad@ear.ro
Web address: www.ear.ro

Peer reviewer: Acad. Constantin POPA

Descrierea CIP a Bibliotecii Naționale a României

Surgical anatomy of the abdomen / ed.: Mircea Beuran, Ionuț Negoi. –
București: Editura Academiei Române, 2016
ISBN 978-973-27-2614-3

I. Beuran, Mircea (ed.)
II. Negoi, Ionuț (ed.)

617.55-089

Editorial Assistants: Monica STANCIU, Doina ARGEȘANU
Computer Editing: Doina STOIA
Cover: Mariana ȘERBĂNESCU

Final proof: 18.04.2016. Format: 16/70 × 100
Proof in sheets: 18
D.C.L. for large libraries: 616.33–089
D.C.L. for small libraries: 61

*To my family for their continuous support
and to my patients for their faith.*

Mircea Beuran

*To my wife Ruxandra Irina and my daughter Ilinca Ioana
for their unconditional love.*

Ionuț Negoi

PREFACE

It is our privilege to introduce a book of surgical anatomy, especially during this time, when classical anatomy with thorough anatomical dissection on cadaveric models has been reduced significantly in medical schools, while the surgeon's needs for anatomical knowledge has continuously increased. In the repertoire of modern general surgery, are included nowadays, trauma and emergency surgery, coloproctology, esophagus and cardia and stomach surgery, surgical oncology, hepato-pancreato-biliary surgery, endocrine surgery, transplant surgery and breast surgery. During the evolution of this speciality, surgical anatomy has experienced new refinements. Throughout this book we intended to fill the gap between all we are learning as students in the pre-clinical years and what we are facing everyday in the operating theaters. We feel that a major strength of this book is integration of embryology details, relevant for the operating surgeon who should develop dissection planes with minimum trauma and blood loss, according to the modern open and minimally invasive surgical principles. The histology data tries to offer to residents and young doctors a tool for better understanding the tissue structures relevant in surgical oncology. Being the first edition of this book, we are aware about the need for further clarification in certain areas and we rely on constructive criticism from our readers. The book is intended for a wide readership across students, residents and general surgery physicians.

We are grateful to our colleagues from the Emergency Hospital of Bucharest, from Surgery, Radiology and Imagistics, Pathology and Gastroenterology Departments who supported us with useful images. Many authors have given us permission to reproduce their figures and detailed acknowledgements are given in the text. The publisher, the Publishing House of the Romanian Academy, enthusiastically supported us with editing of our book and provided us with outstanding assistance.

We hope that this book will not linger on the shelf and will be a constant place to return to for revising anatomy before going into the operating room.

Bucharest, November 2015

Mircea Beuran

Ionuţ Negoi

AUTHORS

Mircea Beuran MD, PhD, FACS, Professor of Surgery, *Carol Davila* University of Medicine and Pharmacy Bucharest, General Surgery Department, Emergency Hospital of Bucharest, No 8 Floreasca Street, 014461, Bucharest, Romania, E-mail: drmirceabeuran@yahoo.com

Ionut Negoi, MD, PhD, Senior Lecturer of Surgery, *Carol Davila* University of Medicine and Pharmacy Bucharest, General Surgery Department, Emergency Hospital of Bucharest, No 8 Floreasca Street, 014461, Bucharest, Romania, E-mail: negoiionut@gmail.com

Alexandru Runcanu, MD, PhD, General Surgery Department, Emergency Hospital of Bucharest, No 8 Floreasca Street, 014461, Bucharest, Romania

Sorin Hostiuc MD, PhD, Lecturer, *Carol Davila* University of Medicine and Pharmacy, Dept of Legal Medicine and Bioethics, Bucharest, No 9 Vitan Barzeşti Street, 042122, Bucharest, Romania. E-mail: soraer@gmail.com

Ruxandra Irina Negoi MD, PhD, Assistant Professor of Anatomy, *Carol Davila* University of Medicine and Pharmacy Bucharest, Anatomy Department, No 8 Eroilor Sanitari Street, 050511, Bucharest, Romania, E-mail: negoiruxandra@gmail.com

Sorin Paun MD, PhD, Senior Lecturer of Surgery, *Carol Davila* University of Medicine and Pharmacy Bucharest, General Surgery Department, Emergency Hospital of Bucharest, No 8 Floreasca Street, 014461, Bucharest, Romania, E-mail: drspaun@yahoo.com

Valentin Enache, MD, Pathology Department, Emergency Hospital of Bucharest, No 8 Floreasca Street, 014461, Bucharest, Romania, E-mail: valienache@rocketmail.com

Bogdan Stoica, MD, PhD student, General Surgery Department, Emergency Hospital of Bucharest, No 8 Floreasca Street, 014461, Bucharest, Romania, E-mail: stoicabogdan85@yahoo.com

Monica Popiel, MD, Radiology and Imagistics Department, Emergency Hospital of Bucharest, No 8 Floreasca Street, 014461, Bucharest, Romania

Daniela Stan, MD, Radiology and Imagistics Department, Emergency Hospital of Bucharest, No 8 Floreasca Street, 014461, Bucharest, Romania

Mihaela Vartic MD, PhD, Anesthesia and Intensive Care Unit, Emergency Hospital of Bucharest, No 8 Floreasca Street, 014461, Bucharest, Romania, Email: mvartic@gmail.com

Ioan Tanase, MD, PhD student, General Surgery Department, Emergency Hospital of Bucharest, No 8 Floreasca Street, 014461, Bucharest, Romania, E-mail: ionatanase@gmail.com

Regina Kirby, *Carol Davila* University of Medicine and Pharmacy Bucharest, E-mail: reginakirby@ymail.com.

Acknowledgment: *The authors would like to thank Regina Kirby for language editing and proofreading of the manuscript.*

CONTENTS

ABBREVIATIONS

AJCC	American Joint Committee on Cancer
APUD cells	Amine precursor uptake and decarboxylation cells
CME	Complete mesocolic excision
CT	Computed Tomography
CVL	Central vascular ligation
ELAPE	Extralevator abdominoperineal excision
EMT	Epithelial to Mesenchymal Transition
ERCP	Endoscopic Retrograde Cholangiopancreatography
FIGO	The International Federation of Gynecology and Obstretics
FJA	First jenunal artery
GIST	Gastrointestinal Stromal Tumors
HCC	Hepatocellular carcinoma
LHA	Left hepatic artery
IVC	Inferior Vena Cava
IPDA	Inferior pancreaticoduodenal artery
MET	Mesenchymal to epithelial transition
MRCP	Magnetic Resonance Cholangiopancreatography
MRI	Magnetic Resonance Imaging
PD	Pancreaticoduodenectomy
PV	Portal vein
RHA	Right hepatic artery
SMA	Superior mesenteric artery
SMV	Superior mesenteric vein

SECTION I – THE ABDOMINAL WALL

An education in medicine involves both learning and learning how;
the student cannot effectively know, unless he knows how.

Abraham Flexner

CHAPTER 1

ANATOMY OF THE ANTEROLATERAL ABDOMINAL WALL

MIRCEA BEURAN, IONUȚ NEGOI

A thorough understanding of the abdominal wall anatomy is of paramount importance for all abdominal surgeons. Every procedure requires access into the abdomen and its closure at the end.

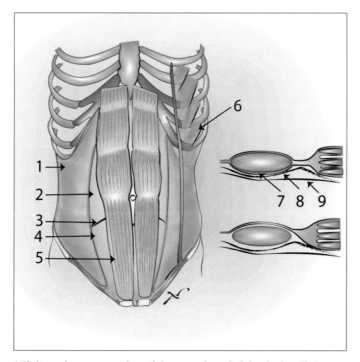

Figure 1 Schematic representation of the anterolateral abdominal wall. 1 – transversus abdominis muscle, 2 – posterior layer of the rectus sheath, 3 – arcuate line of Douglas, 4 – anterior parietal peritoneum below the arcuate line, 5 – rectus abdominis muscle, 6 – external oblique muscle. Transversal sections through the rectus sheath, above the Douglas's arcuate line (7 – posterior layer of the rectus sheath, 8 – transversalis fascia, 9 – anterior peritoneum) and below the arcuate line (it can be observed the absence of the posterior layer of the rectus sheath) (Personal courtesy IN).

An appropriate approach has direct impact on the operating field and intraoperative complications, while closure of the abdominal incisions strongly correlates with the long-term morbidities, quality of life and healthcare costs. The anterolateral abdominal wall consists of the rectus abdominis muscles with their fascial system (rectus sheath), anteriorly, and external oblique, internal oblique and transversus abdominis muscles, laterally. The rectus sheath is an aponeurotic system which encloses the rectus abdominis muscles. In the upper two thirds of the rectus abdominis muscles, the rectus sheath has an anterior and posterior layer. The anterior sheath is composed of the external oblique aponeurosis and the posterior sheath by the transversus abdominis aponeurosis. The aponeurosis of the internal oblique muscles divides into an anterior lamina, which joins the external oblique aponeurosis, and a posterior lamina, which passes posterior to the rectus abdominis muscles and fuses with the transversus abdominis aponeurosis. The aponeuroses which form the rectus sheath join in the midline at the level of the linea alba. The linea alba is a fibrous structure, spanning from the xiphoid process to the pubic symphysis. Its width is wider above the umbilicus and narrower below. In the lower third, the rectus sheath has only an anterior component, from the aponeuroses of all three lateral muscles. The inferior edge of the posterior lamina of the rectus sheath is termed the arcuate line of Douglas. Deep to these muscles and fasciae, the anterolateral abdominal wall includes the transversalis fascia and the parietal peritoneum.

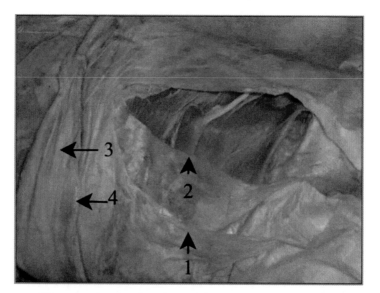

Figure 2. Dissection on a cadaveric model of the anterolateral abdominal wall revealing the anterior parietal peritoneum (1), transversalis fascia (2), median umbilical ligament (urachus) (3), and the medial umbilical ligament (obliterated umbilical arteries) (4) (Image courtesy of IN).

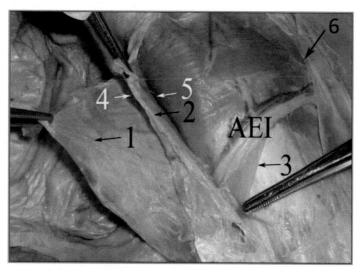

Figure 3. Dissection on a cadaveric model of the anterolateral abdominal wall revealing the anterior parietal peritoneum (1), transversalis fascia with its posterior (2) and anterior layers (3) bounding a vascular space (4) for inferior epigastric vessels (AEI). 5 – Bogros space, 6 – arcuate line of Douglas or the inferior edge of the posterior layer of the rectus sheath (Image courtesy of IN).

When a surgeon chooses an abdominal incision she or he should consider the necessity of appropriate exposure of the operating field, certainty of the diagnosis, potential for major intraoperative bleeding, postoperative pain and cosmetic results.

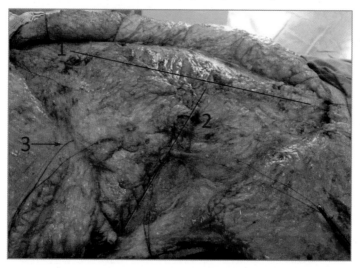

Figure 4. Intraoperative view of a combined J shape incision with midline laparotomy (1 and 2) for a patient with a segment 6 and 7 liver metastasis and giant incisional hernia two years after a low anterior resection for rectal cancer. 3 – transparietal "U" shape sutures used to fix the onlay mesh (Image from personal collection of IN).

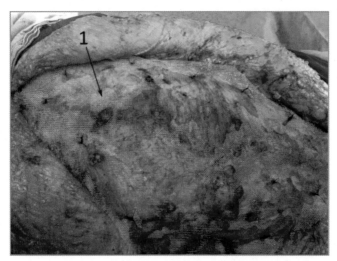

Figure 5. Intraoperative view of a combined J shape incision with midline laparotomy for a patient with a segment 6 and 7 liver metastasis and giant incisional hernia two years after a low anterior resection for rectal cancer. 1 – the onlay polypropylene mesh (Image from personal collection of IN).

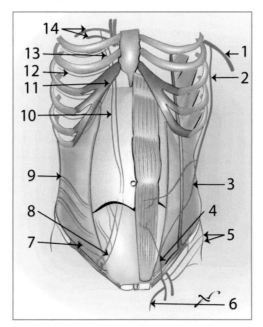

Figure 6. Schematic representation of vascular supply of the anterolateral abdominal wall. 1 – axillary vein, 2 – lateral thoracic vein, 3 – thoracoepigastric vein, 4 – superficial epigastric vein, 5 – superficial circumflex iliac vessels, 6 – great saphenous vein, 7 – deep circumflex iliac vessels, 8 – inferior epigastric vessels, 9 – subcostal vessels, 10 – superior epigastric vessels, 11 – musculophrenic vessels, 12 – anterior intercostal vessels, 13 – internal thoracic vessels, 14 – subclavian vessels (Personal courtesy IN).

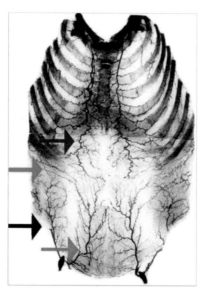

Figure 7. Vasculature of the deep tissues of the anterior abdominal wall demonstrated on fresh cadaveric injection. Red arrow 1/4 deep inferior epigastric artery. Black arrow 1/4 deep circumflex iliac artery. Green arrow 1/4 intercostal arteries. Purple arrow 1/4 deep superior epigastric artery [Figure reproduced with permission from John Wiley and Sons, from W.M. Rozen, M.W. Ashton, G.I. Taylor. Reviewing the vascular supply of the anterior abdominal wall: Redefining anatomy for increasingly refined surgery. Clinical Anatomy, 21, 89–98, 2008 (Rozen, Ashton and Taylor, 2008)].

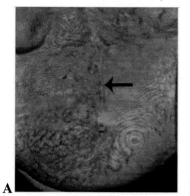
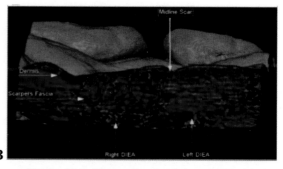

Figure 8. A: Computed tomographic angiogram (CTA) with volume rendered technique (VRT) reformat, performed on the cadaveric specimen. A large midline scar is evident (black arrow). The arterial filling of the right superficial arterial system (green vessels) is evident, terminating at the level of the scar. There is no filling of the left superficial arterial system. B: Axial view of the cadaveric computed tomographic angiogram (CTA) with volume rendered technique (VRT). Filling of the deep inferior epigastric arteries (DIEAs) bilaterally is shown (green vessels), as is filling of the right superficial arterial system. The left superficial arterial system is not filled to the left of the scar [Figure reproduced with permission from John Wiley and Sons, from Warren M. Rozen, Emilio Garcia-Tutor, Alberto Alonso-Burgos, Russell J. Corlett, G. Ian Taylor, Mark W. Ashton. The effect of anterior abdominal wall scars on the vascular anatomy of the abdominal wall: A cadaveric and clinical study with clinical implications. Clinical Anatomy. 22, 815–823, 2009 (Rozen *et al.*, 2009)].

CHAPTER 2
ABDOMINAL INCISIONS

If you want a thing done well, do it yourself.
Napoleon Bonaparte

MIRCEA BEURAN, IONUȚ NEGOI

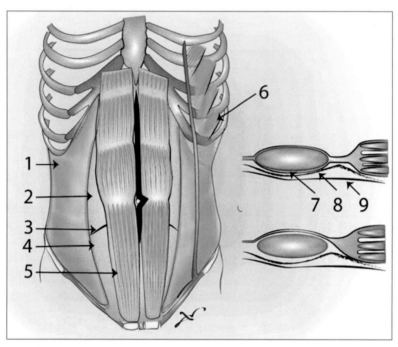

Figure 9. Schematic representation of the midline laparotomy. It offers rapid access to the peritoneal cavity (e.g., exploratory laparotomy for trauma) and a large access, especially when the diagnosis is uncertain. The midline laparotomy produces minimal blood loss and nerve injuries, is appropriate for repeated celiotomies, but compared to transverse incisions is associated with a higher risk of incisional hernia. Laterally, transverse oblique extension of the incision can be added when necessary. 1 – transversus abdominis muscle, 2 – posterior layer of the rectus sheath, 3 – arcuate line of Douglas, 4 – anterior parietal peritoneum below the arcuate line, 5 – rectus abdominis muscle, 6 – external oblique muscle. Transverse sections through the rectus sheath, above the Douglas's arcuate line (7 – posterior layer of the rectus sheath, 8 – transversalis fascia, 9 – anterior peritoneum) and below the arcuate line (it can be observed the absence of the posterior layer of the rectus sheath) (Personal courtesy IN).

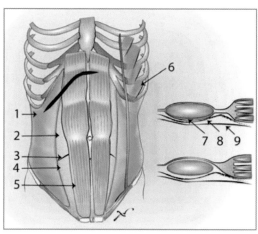

Figure 10. Schematic representation of the right subcostal laparotomy, preferred for open cholecystectomy and common bile duct exploration. 1 – transversus abdominis muscle, 2 – posterior layer of the rectus sheath, 3 – arcuate line of Douglas, 4 – anterior parietal peritoneum below the arcuate line, 5 – rectus abdominis muscle, 6 – external oblique muscle. Transverse sections through the rectus sheath, above the Douglas's arcuate line (7 – posterior layer of the rectus sheath, 8 – transversalis fascia, 9 – anterior peritoneum) and below the arcuate line (it can be observed the absence of the posterior layer of the rectus sheath) (Personal courtesy IN).

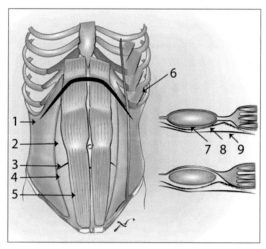

Figure 11. Schematic representation of the bisubcostal (chevron) laparotomy, useful for hepato-bilio-pancreatic procedures. The transverse incision should be done around three centimeters below the costal margin. The exposure may be improved by adding a vertical midline extension ('Mercedes' star incision). 1 – transversus abdominis muscle, 2 – posterior layer of the rectus sheath, 3 – arcuate line of Douglas, 4 – anterior parietal peritoneum below the arcuate line, 5 – rectus abdominis muscle, 6 – external oblique muscle. Transverse sections through the rectus sheath, above the Douglas's arcuate line (7 – posterior layer of the rectus sheath, 8 – transversalis fascia, 9 – anterior peritoneum) and below the arcuate line (it can be observed, the absence of the posterior layer of the rectus sheath) (Image courtesy of IN).

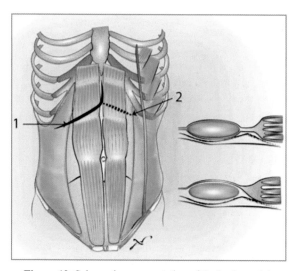

Figure 12. Schematic representation of the hockey stick
(1) with mercedes extension (2) laparotomy, useful for complex
hepato-bilio-pancreatic procedures (Image courtesy of IN).

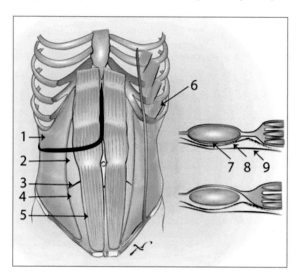

Figure 13. Schematic representation of the 'J shape' laparotomy, popularized by Masatoshi Makuuchi, most frequently used for surgical resections on the right hemiliver. It offers particularly good exposure of the right hepatic vein – inferior vena cava junction. Can be extended into the right thorax through the seventh intercostal space. 1 – transversus abdominis muscle, 2 – posterior layer of the rectus sheath, 3 – arcuate line of Douglas, 4 – anterior parietal peritoneum below the arcuate line, 5 – rectus abdominis muscle, 6 – external oblique muscle. Transverse sections through the rectus sheath, above the Douglas's arcuate line (7 – posterior layer of the rectus sheath, 8 – transversalis fascia, 9 – anterior peritoneum) and below the arcuate line (it can be observed, the absence of the posterior layer of the rectus sheath) (Image courtesy of IN).

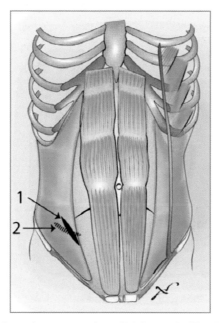

Figure 14. Schematic representation of McBurney's (1) or Rockey-Davis (2) incisions, ideal for open appendectomy (Image courtesy of IN).

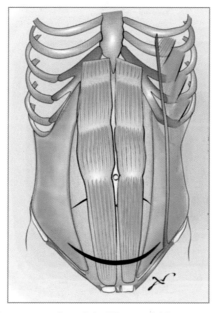

Figure 15. Schematic representation of the Pfannenstiel laparotomy (when the muscular layer is sectioned through a vertical incision, at the level of the linea alba) or a Maylard laparotomy (when the rectus abdominis muscles are sectioned transversally, in the same plane as the skin) (Image courtesy of IN).

SECTION II – THE PERITONEUM

It is not birth, marriage or death which is the most important time in your life, but Gastrulation.

Lewis Wolpert

CHAPTER 3

EMBRYOLOGY

RUXANDRA IRINA NEGOI

The development of the serous membranes, such as pleura, serous pericardium and peritoneum, and of the serous cavities of the body are related to the embryologic development of the intraembryonic mesoderm (Skandalakis *et al.*, 2004). This is the third layer of the human embryo, and appears at the third week of gestation after a process termed gastrulation (Negoi *et al.*, 2010). Towards the end of the third week (Sadler, 2009), the mesoderm is located lateral to the notochord, along the length of the embryo, and is divided into three components:
- The paraxial mesoderm, forming the somites.
- The intermediate mesoderm, giving rise to nephrotomes.
- The lateral mesoderm, which forms the body cavity, including the serosa.
The lateral mesoderm is then cleaved into two layers:
- Parietal or somatic layer, which accompanies the ectodermal embryonic layer, and gives rise to the serous parietal membranes of the trunk, such as the parietal peritoneum, the pleura and the pericardium.
- Visceral or splanchnic layer, which accompanies the embryonic endoderm. The endoderm will give rise to the mucosal layer of the digestive tract, while the visceral layer of the lateral mesoderm will contribute to the submucosal, muscular and serosal layers of the gastrointestinal tract. From the visceral layer of the lateral mesoderm will develop also the visceral pleura and the pericardium.

The anatomical space located between the two layers is termed the primitive body cavity. Through the development of the diaphragm, the pleural cavities are separated by the peritoneal space (Negoi *et al.*, 2010).

The connection between the somatic and visceral mesoderm is made by mesenteries (Moore and Persaud, 2008). The primitive gut is related to the embryonic trunk by two such mesenteries, termed:
- Dorsal mesentery – over the entire length of the primitive gut. The arteries which supply the primitive gut are found between the two layers of the dorsal mesentery: the celiac artery for the foregut, the superior mesenteric artery for the midgut and the inferior mesenteric artery for the hindgut (Moore and Persaud, 2008).
- Ventral mesentery – shorter and found only at the level of the distal foregut (primordium of the stomach and proximal part of the duodenum) (Sadler, 2009).

CHAPTER 4

ANATOMY

MIRCEA BEURAN, IONUŢ NEGOI

The peritoneum is a serous membrane which covers the abdominal cavity and its contained viscera, with a mean surface of 14323.62 ± 824 cm^2 (Albanese *et al.*, 2009).

Table 1
Pattern of cancer cell dissemination in peritoneal carcinomatosis (Coccolini *et al.*, 2013)

Pattern of spread	Molecular mechanisms	Biology of the tumor cells	Primary tumor
Random proximal distribution	Early implantation via adherence of molecules on the surface of cancer cells.	Moderate and high grade cancers	Adenocarcinoma and carcinoid of the appendix Non-mucinous colorectal cancer Gastric cancer Serous ovarian cancer
Complete redistribution	No adhesion close to the primary tumor.	Low biological aggressiveness	Pseudomyxoma peritonei Diffuse malignant mesothelioma
Widespread cancer distribution	Mucous secretion which prevents cell adhesion	Aggressive tumors	Mucinous ovarian cancer Mucinous colorectal cancer

It can be divided into a parietal layer, lining the abdominal cavity and a visceral layer, covering the abdominal viscera. The two peritoneal layers are continuous, and the peritoneal cavity forms between them (Ba-Ssalamah *et al.*, 2009). Normally, the peritoneal cavity contains a small volume of peritoneal fluid (50–100 ml), which slightly increases at the midpoint of the menstrual cycle in females (Blackburn and Stanton, 2014). The role of this peritoneal fluid is to moisten the viscera, facilitating sliding between themselves and against the walls of the abdominal cavity.

The visceral peritoneum is quite thin and highly adherent to the covered abdominal organ. It can not be surgically separated from the covered organ. The visceral peritoneum has a common blood supply and innervation with the covered abdominal organs. Having an autonomous innervation, its irritation in various abdominal pathologies generates a dull and imprecisely defined pain. The parietal peritoneum is thick and loosely adherent to the abdominal wall, from which it can be surgically detached. The parietal peritoneum has a common innervation and vascular supply with the abdominal wall. Due to its somatic innervation, its impairment by different abdominal pathologies gives an acute, well circumscribed pain (Negoi *et al.*, 2010).

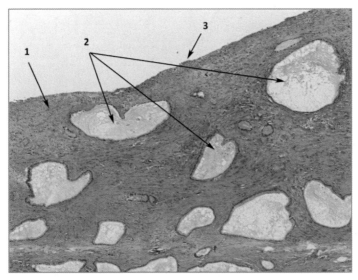

Figure 16. Hematoxylin and Eosin staining using 50 × objective of peritoneum with metastasis of adenocarcinoma (2): 1 – peritumoral fibrous tissue, 3 – mesothelial cells (Image courtesy of VE, used with permission).

PERITONEAL EXTENSIONS

The peritoneum and its adherences to the abdominal organs gives rise to anatomical structures named ligaments, mesenteries, and coalescence fascia.

The peritoneal ligaments connect two abdominal organs, or an abdominal organ to the abdominal wall. For example, the gastrocolic ligament is located between the stomach and the transverse colon, and the splenorenal ligament connects the spleen with the left kidney. The mesenteries are anatomical structures that connect the abdominal organs to the posterior abdominal wall. They are longer, and confer mobility to the intraperitoneal organs. For example, the transverse mesocolon connects the transverse colon to the posterior abdominal wall, while the small bowel mesentery connects the jejunum and the ileum to the posterior abdominal wall.

The coalescence fascia may be found at the level of the secondary retroperitoneal organs, between them and the posterior abdominal wall. For example, the Treitz pancreaticoduodenal fascia is found posterior to the duodenum and pancreas, and the Toldt I fascia is located posterior to the ascending colon.

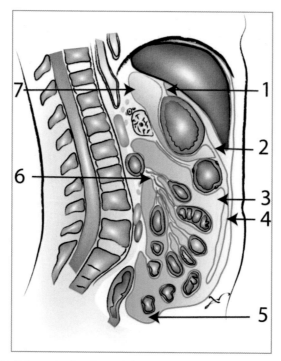

Figure 17. Schematic drawing of the lateral view of the peritoneal space:
1 – gastrohepatic ligament, 2 – gastrocolic ligament, 3 – inframesocolic space
of the abdominal peritoneal cavity, 4 – greater omentum, 5 – Douglas pouch,
6 – mesenterium, 7 – omental bursa (Figure courtesy of IN).

DIVISION OF THE ABDOMINAL CAVITY

Related to the anatomical distribution of the peritoneum, the abdominal
cavity may be divided into a peritoneal and an extraperitoneal space. The extraperitoneal space may be further divided into the preperitoneal, retroperitoneal and
pelvis-subperitoneal spaces. The peritoneal cavity may be divided into abdominal
and pelvic spaces, the limit being the upper pelvic brim.

THE ABDOMINAL PERITONEAL SPACE

The abdominal peritoneal space may be divided for educational purposes,
into greater and lesser peritoneal cavities.

This subdivision of the abdominal peritoneal cavity occurs during the
intrauterine life, by right side rotation of the primitive gut and its ventral and dorsal
mesenteries.

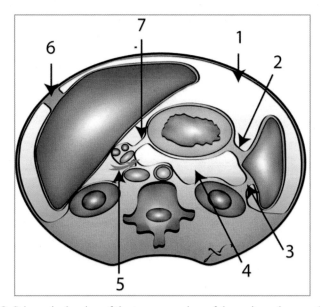

Figure 18. Schematic drawing of the transverse view of the peritoneal space: 1 – greater peritoneal cavity, 2 – gastrosplenic ligament, 3 – splenorenal ligament, 4 – omental bursa or lesser sac, 5 – Winslow orifice (Figure courtesy of IN).

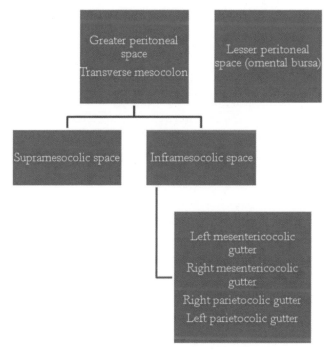

Figure 19. Anatomical division of the abdominal cavity.

THE PELVIC PERITONEAL SPACE

The peritoneum covering the pelvic organs, gives rise to the lowest space of the peritoneal cavity, where most of the pathological abdominal conditions may be found. In the male pelvis, the peritoneum covers the rectum and the urinary bladder, forming the recto-vesical pouch. In women, the peritoneum forms the recto-uterine or Douglas pouch and the vesico-uterine pouch.

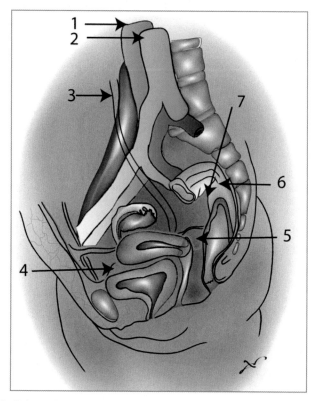

Figure 20. Schematic drawing of the sagittal view of the pelvic peritoneal space: 1 – inferior vena cava, 2 – aorta, 3 – right ureter, 4 – vesico-uterine pouch, 5 – recto-uterine or Douglas pouch, 6 – rectum, 7 – visceral peritoneum (Figure courtesy of IN).

SECTION III – THE DIAPHRAGM

A blind man works on wood the same way as a surgeon on the body, when he's ignorant of anatomy.

Guy de Chauliac

CHAPTER 5

EMBRYOLOGY

RUXANDRA IRINA NEGOI

The embryological development of the diaphragm involves (Moore and Persaud, 2008; Sadler, 2009):

The septum transversum

The pleuroperitoneal membranes

The dorsal mesentery of the esophagus

The somites at cervical segments three to five.

Muscular ingrowth from the lateral body walls.

The septum transversum is the primordium of the central tendon of the diaphragm. The pleuroperitoneal membranes form the lateral area of the diaphragm (Negoi *et al.*, 2010).

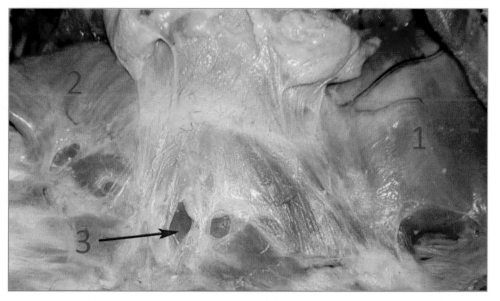

Figure 21. Dissection on a cadaveric model, revealing the left (1) and right (2) hemidiaphragm. The liver can be observed through the Larrey-Morgagni space (3) (Image personal courtesy of SH, IN).

The dorsal mesentery of the esophagus gives rise to the lumbar part of the diaphragm.

The muscular component of the diaphragm, with its origin in somites from the cervical segments, explains the motor and sensory innervation of the diaphragm, through the phrenic nerves (originating from the C3-C5 spinal cord) (Sadler, 2009).

The costal area of the diaphragm receives sensory fibers from the lower intercostal nerves, due to its embryological origin in the lateral body walls (Moore and Persaud, 2008).

All these parts of the diaphragm, with different embryological origins will merge, first on the right side and then on the left. Congenital diaphragmatic hernias occur through defects in the fusion process of different parts of the diaphragm (Sadler, 2009). The diaphragmatic hernias may be:

Posterolateral – through lack of fusion between of the pleuroperitoneal membranes and the other three parts of the diaphragm. These are termed the Bochdalek's hernia and occur in 85–90% of cases on the left side.

Retrosternal – appears through the sternocostal triangle of Morgagni. Through this diaphragmatic defect, abdominal viscera may herniate into the pericardial sac or the heart can descend into the peritoneal cavity.

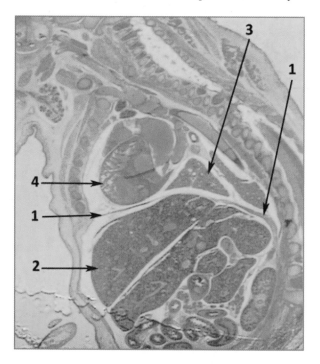

Figure 22. Sagittal section through the body of a rat embryo revealing the diaphragm (1), the liver (2), the lung (3), and the heart (4) (Figure courtesy of RIN).

Increasing evidence supports that the diaphragm mainly develops from (a) the transverse septum that give rise to the floor of the pericardial cavity; (b) a posthepatic mesenchymal plate that develops in close relationship with the underlying liver; (c) the pleuroperitoneal fold, that contributes to the lateral margins of the diaphragm; and (d) the pleuroperitoneal canal, that is closed by the neighboring organs and the ingrowth of the posthepatic mesenchyme (Babiuk *et al.*, 2003; Mayer, Metzger & Kluth, 2011). If the normal embryological development of this posthepatic mesenchymal plate, which contribute mainly to the growing part of the diaphragm, is impaired a diaphragmatic congenital hernia occurs (Mayer, Metzger & Kluth, 2011). Significant morbidity and mortality in newborns with congenital diaphragmatic hernia is due to the associated pulmonary hypoplasia and persistent pulmonary hypertension (Keijzer & Puri, 2010; Greer, 2013).

CHAPTER 6

ANATOMY

MIRCEA BEURAN, IONUȚ NEGOI

The diaphragm is a muscular, dome-shaped anatomical structure, that separates the thoracic from the abdominal cavity. At the end of expiration the right diaphragm is projected at the level of the fifth rib in the midclavicular line, while the left diaphragm is projected at the fifth intercostal space in the midclavicular line (Negoi *et al.*, 2010).

ORIGIN AND INSERTION OF THE DIAPHRAGM

The diaphragm has a central area, termed the central tendon, from which the muscular fibers radiate in all directions, to their peripheral origin.

The origins of the diaphragm may be divided into three areas: a lumbar, a costal and a sternal one. The lumbar origin is represented by the two crura of the diaphragm, together with the medial and lateral arcuate ligaments. The crura of the diaphragm are muscular and tendinous structures, originating from the anterior surface of the lumbar vertebral bodies, intervertebral discs, and the anterior longitudinal ligament. The right crus is thicker and longer, originating from the L1-L4 vertebrae. The left crus is thinner and shorter, originating from the L1-L3 vertebrae.

The medial tendinous fibers from the two crura cross the midline, anterior to the aorta, forming the median arcuate ligament. The medial arcuate ligament expands from the L2 vertebral body to the L1 transverse process, arching over the psoas muscle. The lateral arcuate ligament expands from the transverse process of the L1 vertebra to the twelfth rib, arching over the quadratus lumborum muscle.

The costal origin of the diaphragm is on the inner surface of the lowest six ribs. The sternal origin is on the posterior surface of the xiphoid process.

Observed form the thorax, the central tendon of the diaphragm has a three-lobed clover shape, with an anterior, a left and a right lobe.

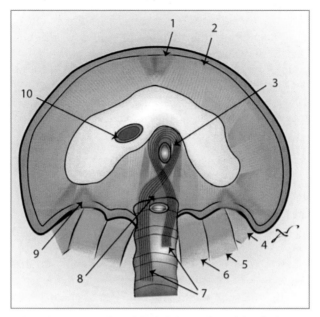

Figure 23. Schematic representation of the inferior surface of the diaphragm: 1 – Larrey-Morgagni's sternocostal triangle, 2 – costal origin of the diaphragm, 3 – esophageal hiatus of the diaphragm, 4 – transversus abdominis muscle, 5 – quadratus lumborum muscle, 6 – psoas muscle, 7 – lumbar origin of the diaphragm, 8 – aortic hiatus, 9 – lumbocostal triangle of Bochadelck, 10 – caval opening (Figure courtesy of IN).

THE DIAPHRAGMATIC HIATUSES

The esophageal hiatus is an oval-shaped opening, projecting at the level of the T10 vertebra. It is formed by muscular fibers, with their origin on the right and left diaphragmatic crura. The esophagus passes through the hiatus together with the anterior and posterior vagal trunks, the esophageal arteries, veins and lymphatic vessels. The hiatal hernia represents a protrusion of the stomach and other abdominal organs, in the mediastinum, through the esophageal hiatus. The most common types are sliding, paraesophageal and mixed hiatal hernias.

The aortic hiatus is bound posteriorly by the vertebral column, laterally by the diaphragmatic crura, and anteriorly by the median arcuate ligament. It is projected at the level of the T12 vertebra, and contains the aorta and the thoracic duct. In 10%–24% of people the median arcuate ligament inserts at a lower level, crossing the anterior surface of the celiac artery (Lindner and Kemprud, 1971). In some of these individuals, the proximal segment of the celiac artery is compressed (Delis *et al.*, 2007).

The inferior vena cava hiatus is located between the anterior and the right leaflets of the central tendon of the diaphragm, projecting at the level of the T8-T9 vertebrae. The walls of the inferior vena cava are adherent to its diaphragmatic hiatus. Thus, during inspiration, the diaphragm contracts, the hiatus expands and the blood flow through the vena cava is increased.

Besides the major hiatuses of the diaphragm, there are also minor orifices, for smaller anatomical structures, like the greater and lesser splanchnic nerves, which traverse the pillars of the diaphragm; the lumbar sympathetic trunks and the ascending lumbar veins, beneath the medial arcuate ligament.

VASCULAR SUPPLY OF THE DIAPHRAGM

The superior surface of the diaphragm receives its arterial supply from the superior phrenic arteries branching off from the thoracic aorta, the musculophrenic and pericardiacophrenic arteries branching off from the internal thoracic arteries, and the lowest sixth intercostal arteries. On the inferior surface, the diaphragm receives its arterial supply through the two inferior phrenic arteries, branching off from the abdominal aorta. The inferior phrenic arteries supply also the adrenal glands through the superior suprarenal arteries. The veins are homonymous to the arteries. The pericardiacophrenic and musculophrenic veins drain into the internal thoracic veins. The inferior right phrenic vein drains into the inferior vena cava. The inferior left phrenic vein usually drains inferiorly into the left adrenal vein and superiorly into the inferior vena cava.

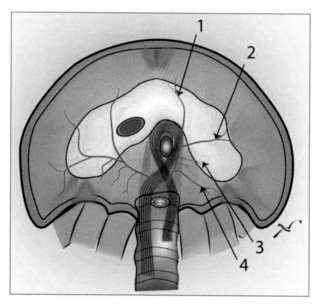

Figure 24. Schematic representation of the inferior surface of the diaphragm with the right and left inferior phrenic arteries. Their branches are: 1 – anterior, 2 – lateral, 3 – posterior, 4 – superior adrenal arteries [Image redrawn by IN after Skandalakis *et al.* (Skandalakis *et al.*, 2004)].

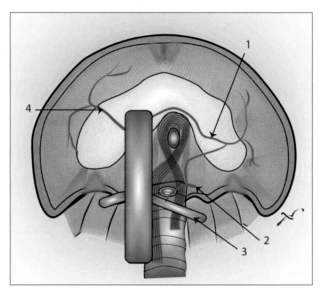

Figure 25. Schematic representation of the inferior surface of the diaphragm with its venous drainage: 1 – left inferior phrenic vein draining superiorly into the inferior vena cava and inferiorly into the central vein of the adrenal gland (2). 3 – left renal vein, 4 – right inferior phrenic vein [Image redrawn by IN after Skandalakis *et al.* (Skandalakis *et al.*, 2004)].

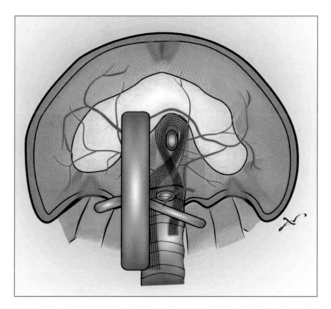

Figure 26. Schematic representation of the inferior surface of the diaphragm with the right and left inferior phrenic arteries and vein [Image redrawn by IN after Skandalakis *et al.* (Skandalakis *et al.*, 2004)].

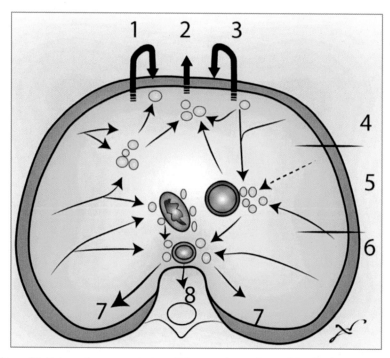

Figure 27. Schematic representation of the superior surface of the diaphragm with its lymphatic drainage: 1 – from the inferior diaphragmatic surface, 2 – to anterior mediastinal lymph nodes, 3 – from the liver, 4 – anterior mediastinal lymph nodes, 5 – middle mediastinal lymph nodes, 6 – posterior mediastinal lymph nodes, 7 – to posterior mediastinal lymph nodes, 8 – to lumbar lymph nodes [Image redrawn by IN after Skandalakis *et al*. (Skandalakis *et al*., 2004)].

The lymphatics of the diaphragm communicate largely superiorly within the thorax and inferiorly within the abdomen. All groups of diaphragmatic lymph nodes are located on its thoracic surface and can be divided into anterior, middle and posterior groups (Skandalakis *et al*., 2004). They drain upward into the parasternal, mediastinal and phrenic lymph nodes. In the abdomen, the lymphatic drainage is to the upper lumbar lymph nodes.

INNERVATION

The motor innervation is through the two phrenic nerves, with their origins in the C3-C5 spinal cord. The sensory innervation is also accomplished by the phrenic nerves, and by the lowest six pairs of intercostal nerves. The right phrenic nerve enters the diaphragm just lateral to the inferior vena cava hiatus, and the left phrenic nerve just lateral to the left border of the heart (Skandalakis *et al.*, 2004). At the level of the diaphragm, the phrenic nerves give off three branches: the anterior, the lateral and the posterior branch.

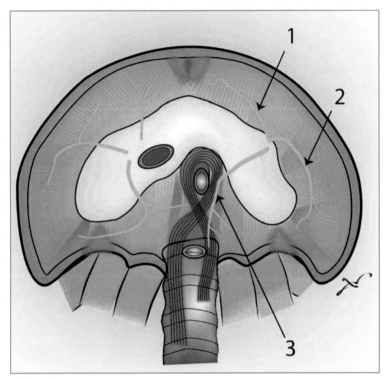

Figure 28. Schematic representation of the inferior surface of the diaphragm with the three branches of the phrenic nerves: anterior (1) lateral (2) and posterior (3) branches (Image redrawn by IN after Skandalakis *et al.* [Skandalakis *et al.*, 2004)].

According to this branching pattern, the surgical incision of the diaphragm should be made circumferential and at its periphery, to avoid the major branches of the phrenic nerve. A radial incision from the periphery to the esophageal hiatus will produce paralysis of the phrenic nerve. Pain with a diaphragmatic origin radiates to the shoulder, especially on the right side, this area being innervated also from the C3-C5 spinal cord, and to the interscapulovertebral region, innervated by the lowest intercostal nerves. Radiated pain into the right shoulder can be from biliary ducts, or the Glisson's capsule of the liver, which also have innervation through the phrenic nerves. The pathological irritation of the phrenic nerve causes hiccups.

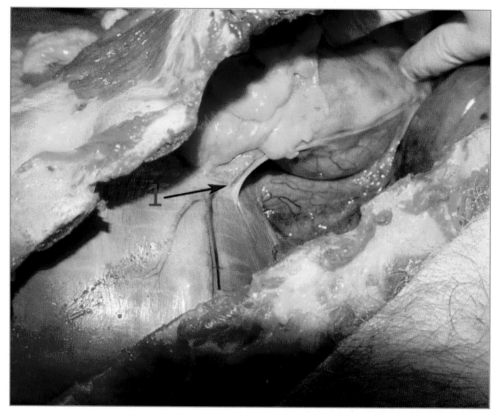

Figure 29. Dissection on a cadaveric model, revealing the left phrenic nerve with the pericardiacophrenic vessels (1) (Image personal courtesy of SH, IN).

CHAPTER 7

HISTOLOGY OF THE DIAPHRAGM

SORIN HOSTIUC, IONUȚ NEGOI

The diaphragm is a muscular and connective tissue structure, including smooth muscles and dense connective tissue, that is continued superiorly with the endothoracic fascia and inferiorly with the endoabdominal, or transversalis fascia. Tumors of the diaphragm are very rare, with only 144 cases of primary tumors reported in the medical literature (Kim & Hofstetter, 2009). The most common benign forms are diaphragmatic cysts and lipoma (Shimizu *et al.*, 1996), but other, like neurofibromas, angiofibromas have been described as well (Sen *et al.*, 2007).

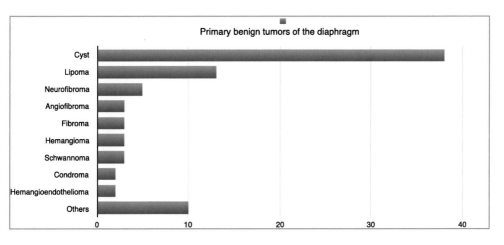

Figure 30. Benign primary tumors of the diaphragm reported in the medical literature [Adapted after (Kim & Hofstetter, 2009)].

The most common malignant neoplastic disease are rhabdomyosarcoma and fibrosarcoma (Mandal, Lee & Salem, 1988; Kim & Hofstetter, 2009), others being only exceptionally described in the scientific literature (chondrosarcoma, leyomio-sarcoma, and so on (Mandal, Lee & Salem, 1988).

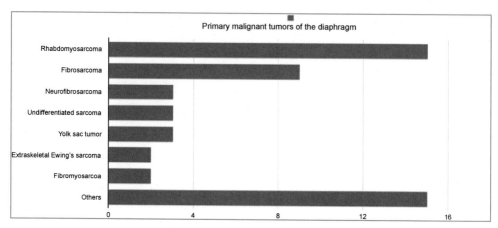

Figure 31. Malignant primary tumors of the diaphragm reported in the medical literature
[Adapted after (Kim & Hofstetter, 2009)].

The majority of tumors of the diaphragm seen in daily clinical practice are metastatic lesions or areas of direct invasion from neighboring malignancies.

The most common metastatic lesions involving the diaphragm are found in patients with ovarian cancer. These patients, with FIGO stage III or IV ovarian cancer, benefit from cytoreductive surgery and hyperthermic intraperitoneal chemotherapy. The residual disease following surgery represents the single most important independent prognostic factor for survival, unrelated to the timing of surgery (Pathiraja, P.N.J., Garruto-Campanile & Tozzi, 2013). The best oncological outcomes are for patients with a R0 resection. In a survey of the Society of Gynecological Oncologists published in 2001, 76.3% of the responders indicated the massive disease on the diaphragm as the main factor precluding optimal cytoreduction, followed only by the portal triad disease (Eisenkop & Spirtos, 2001). In this setting, the surgical efforts to achieve a complete cytoreduction often involve diaphragm stripping or a full-thickness diaphragmatic resection. Thus, the expertise in diaphragm peritonectomy and/or resection is mandatory before starting surgery in patients with ovarian cancer (Kehoe, Eisenhauer & Chi, 2008).

Diaphragmatic resections are also indicated for upper abdominal malignancies with direct invasion of the diaphragm, such as primary or secondary liver tumors, esogastric junction cancers, kidney or adrenal tumors. A propensity-matched analysis of simultaneous diaphragm and liver resection, using data from the American College of Surgeons National Surgical Quality Improvement Program, showed that the need for diaphragm resection was associated with a higher rate of overall (38.5% *vs.* 28.6%, p = 0.048) and major (33.3% *vs.* 23.4%, p = 0.03) complications, with longer operative times (311 *vs.* 247.5 minutes, p < 0.001) and a higher intraoperative blood transfusion rate (33.3% *vs.* 23.4%, p = 0.037) (Li *et al.*, 2013). Yamashita *et al.* evaluated the surgical and oncological outcomes in 27 patients with gross involvement of the diaphragm (13 patients with resection versus 14 patients with blunt dissection) out of 911 patients with hepatocellular carcinoma (HCC) (Yamashita *et al.*, 2011). The authors recommend en bloc resection of the diaphragm in patients with gross diaphragmatic involvement of HCC, since there were no significant differences in short- and long-term surgical impacts, when compared with blunt dissection only. Li *et al.* concluded that simultaneous diaphragm resection during hepatectomy for metastatic colorectal cancer does not significantly influence the preoperative morbidity and mortality despite longer operation times (Li *et al.*, 2012).

SECTION IV – THE ESOPHAGUS

*Where there is love for mankind, there is love
for the art of healing.*

Hippocrates

CHAPTER 8

EMBRYOLOGY

RUXANDRA IRINA NEGOI, MIHAELA VARTIC

THE EMBRYOLOGICAL DEVELOPMENT OF THE DIGESTIVE TRACT□ GENERAL CONSIDERATIONS

Throughout its length, the digestive tract has a similar structure, including mucosa, submucosa, muscularis propria and serosa.

The epithelium of the mucosa and its corresponding glands have an endodermal origin, while the submucosa, muscularis propria and serosa have a mesodermal origin (Moore and Persaud, 2008). Autonomous intramural nervous structures and the APUD cells have their embryological origin in the neural crest cells (Negoi et al., 2010).

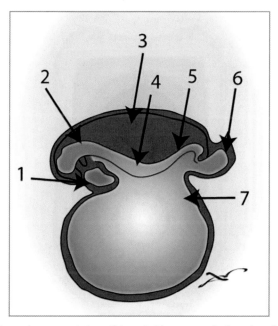

Figure 32. Schematic representation of the primitive gut, sagittal section: 1 – primordium of the heart, 2 – foregut, 3 – amniotic cavity, 4 – midgut, 5 – foregut, 6 – allantois, 7 – yolk sac [Personal courtesy RIN, used with permission of the authors from (Negoi, 2014)].

During the second week of intrauterine life, the endoderm develops on the inferior surface of the embryonic disk. Following the transverse and cephalocaudal embryonic disc folding, the endoderm will be incorporated inside the embryo, giving rise to the primitive gut (Sadler, 2009). The primitive gut is closed at its cranial end, until the third week, by the oropharyngeal membrane. Until the third month of intrauterine life, the distal end of the digestive tract is closed by the cloacal membrane.

The primitive gut is divided into three segments:

The foregut, from the oropharyngeal membrane to distal end of the hepatocystic bud.

The midgut, which starts caudal to the liver bud and extends to the point between the right two thirds and the left third of the transverse colon.

The hindgut, which extends from the left third of the transverse colon to the cloacal membrane.

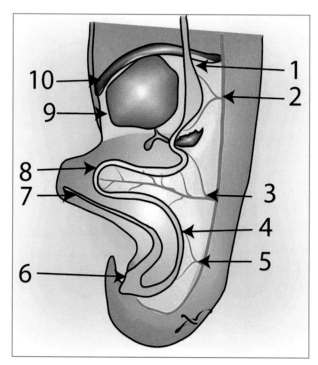

Figure 33. Schematic representation of the primitive gut: 1 – primordium of the stomach, 2 – celiac artery, 3 – superior mesenteric artery, 4 – hindgut, 5 – inferior mesenteric artery, 6 – cloacal membrane, 7 – allantois, 8 – midgut, 9 – primitive ventral mesentery, 10 – septum transversum (Personal courtesy RIN).

The primitive gut is connected to the embryonic body by two mesenteries:

The common dorsal mesentery, which can be found from the lower esophagus to the cloacal membrane.

The ventral mesentery, shorter and only at the level of the distal esophagus, stomach and upper duodenal segment. Its inferior border is located at the middle point of the duodenal loop, next to the origin of the hepatocystic bud.

Through the dorsal mesentery, the gastrointestinal tract receives its arterial blood supply, originating from the dorsal aorta. There are three arterial sources for the primitive gut:

The celiac artery, supplying the foregut.

The superior mesenteric artery, supplying the midgut.

The inferior mesenteric artery, supplying the hindgut.

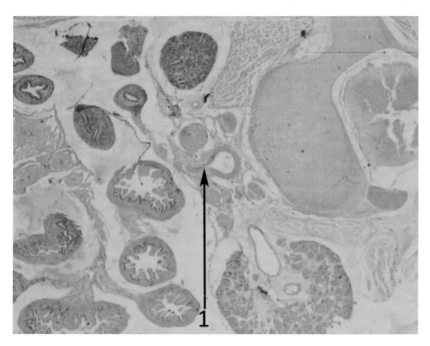

Figure 34. Transverse section through the abdomen of a rat embryo revealing the emergence of the superior mesenteric artery from the abdominal aorta (1) (Figure from personal courtesy of RIN).

The mucosa and the glands of the digestive tract have the following endodermal origin:

From the foregut – the esophagus, stomach and upper half of the duodenum.

From the midgut – the lower half of the duodenum, jejunum, ileum, cecum, vermiform appendix, ascending colon and right two thirds of the transverse colon.

From the hindgut – the left third of the transverse colon, descending colon, sigmoid and the rectum.

EMBRYOLOGICAL DEVELOPMENT OF THE ESOPHAGUS

The esophagus has its embryological origin at the level of the foregut. From the ventral surface of the foregut, in the pharyngeal area will develop the respiratory bud. This will have a caudal development, being delimitated via the tracheoesophageal septum by the foregut (Sadler, 2009). The respiratory bud will give rise to the respiratory system. This common embryological origin may explain congenital esophagotracheal fistula development.

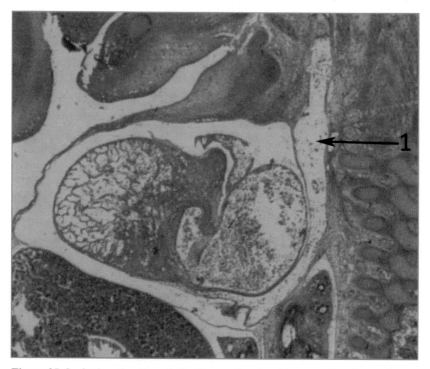

Figure 35. Sagittal section through the thorax of a rat embryo revealing the esophagus (1) (Figure from personal courtesy of RIN).

Early during organ development, due to the shortness of the esophagus, the stomach has a high position. In the latter phases of intrauterine life, the esophagus elongates, due to several factors:

The development of the heart.

The development of the cervical region of the embryo.

The development of the body of the embryo, especially the dorsal wall of the trunk.

The esophageal mucosa and associated ducts and glands are derivatives of the endoderm. The mesoderm forms the lamina propria, muscularis mucosa and the muscular layer (the branchial arches forming the striated muscles and the visceral splanchnic mesoderm forming the smooth muscles) (Lerut *et al.*, 2011). The circular muscular layer develops early in the sixth week, while the longitudinal musculature appears between weeks 9–15. The muscularis mucosa appears during the fourth month. Arteries and veins enter the esophageal wall during the seventh month, while the lymphatics enter during month three – four after birth (Skandalakis *et al.*, 2004).

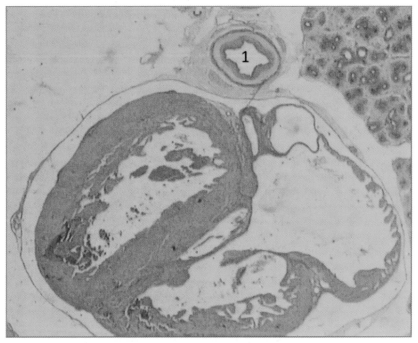

Figure 36. Transverse section through the thorax of a rat embryo revealing the esophagus (1) (Figure from personal courtesy of RIN).

CHAPTER 9

ANATOMY

MIRCEA BEURAN, IONUȚ NEGOI

The esophagus is a 25 cm long and 2 cm wide muscular conduit, with three anatomical regions: a cervical, thoracic and abdominal one. From a surgical point of view the esophagus may be divided according to the tracheal bifurcation into a proximal and a distal segment (Skandalakis *et al.*, 2004).

The esophagus presents three indentations (Lerut *et al.*, 2011):

• The upper esophageal sphincter, located 15–17 cm from the incisor teeth. The upper esophageal sphincter is a true anatomic sphincter, represented by the cricopharyngeus muscle.

• An indentation due to the left main bronchus and the aortic arch, located 25 cm from the incisors.

• The lower esophageal sphincter, located 38–40 cm from the incisors, is a physiological sphincter, represented by a high pressure zone.

Table 2
Anatomical division of the esophagus according to the TNM staging manual (Edge *et al.*, 2010)

Anatomical parts	Arbitrary division into three parts	Anatomical boundaries	Distance from incisors (cm)
Cervical	Upper	Pharynx to sternal notch	15–20
Thoracic		Sternal notch to azygos vein	20–25
	Middle	Azygos vein to inferior pulmonary vein	25–30
	Lower	Inferior pulmonary vein to esophagogastric junction	30–40
Abdominal	Esophagogastric junction	Esophagogastric junction to 5 cm below esophagogastric junction	40–45

According to the seventh edition of the TNM staging manual, the esophago-gastric junction and the proximal 5 cm of the stomach are included in the same class as esophageal cancers (Edge *et al.*, 2010).

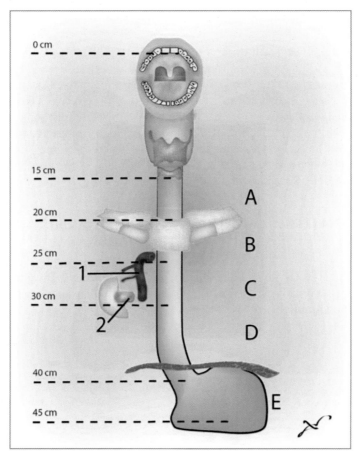

Figure 37. Schematic representation of the anatomical parts of the esophagus and their relationship with surrounding structures: A – cervical, B – upper thoracic, C – middle thoracic, D – lower thoracic, and E – abdominal esophagus. 1 – azygos vein, 2 – right inferior pulmonary vein. A + B = upper esophagus, C = middle esophagus, D + E = lower esophagus (Image courtesy of IN).

In Western literature the cancers of the esophagogastric junction are divided according to Siewert's classification (Rüdiger Siewert *et al.*, 2000):
- Type I: cancers with their center located within 5 cm to 1 cm proximal to the esophagogastric junction.
- Type II: cancer with their center located within 1 cm proximal to 2 cm distal from the esophagogastric junction.
- Type III: cancers with their center located within 2 cm to 5 cm distal to the esophagogastric junction.

According to the Nishi's classification, the Japanese literature defines as cancer of the esophagogastric junction, tumors with their center 2 cm proximal to and distal from the esophagogastric junction (Japan Esophageal Society, 2009).

Cancers of the abdominal esophagus are thus included in cancers of the esophago-gastric junction.

The abdominal segment of the esophagus is 1.5–2.5 cm in length. Having the incisor teeth as an anatomical landmark, the cardiac orifice is located at a mean distance of 44 cm. The upper limit of the abdominal esophagus is represented by its diaphragmatic hiatus, projected at the level of the T10 vertebra. The inferior limit of the abdominal esophagus is located on the esophagogastric junction, or the cardiac orifice. The anatomical projection of the cardiac orifice is anteriorly on the seventh rib cartilage and posteriorly on the T11 vertebra. Inside the lumen, the esophago-gastric junction is marked by the Z-line, a sudden change of the esophageal mucosa with the gastric one (Negoi *et al.*, 2010).

THE ANATOMICAL RELATIONSHIP OF THE ABDOMINAL ESOPHAGUS WITH THE DIAPHRAGM

The esophageal hiatus of the diaphragm has a close anatomic relationship with the pleura superiorly, with the phrenoesophageal membrane in the middle and with the peritoneum inferiorly.

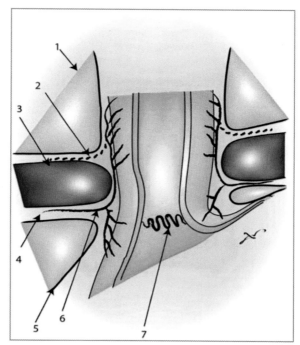

Figure 38. Schematic representation of the esophageal hiatus: 1 – mediastinal pleura, 2 – endothoracic fascia, 3 – diaphragm, 4 – endoabdominal or transversalis fascia, 5 – parietal peritoneum from the inferior surface of the diaphragm, 6 – Laimer-Bertelli's phrenoesophageal membrane, 7 – Z-line (Personal courtesy IN).

Laimer-Bertelli's phrenoesophageal membrane continues the endoabdominal transversalis fascia, from the inferior surface of the diaphragm. This phrenoesophageal membrane has an ascending and a descending lamina. The ascending lamina has a truncated cone shape, and surrounds the esophagus circumferentially, 2 cm above the diaphragm. The descending lamina surrounds the abdominal esophagus. This anatomical structure loses its function in patients with hiatal hernia. The main function of the phrenoesophageal membrane is to seal the esophageal hiatus, maintaining the pressure difference between the thorax and the abdomen, while respecting mobility during respiration.

THE ANATOMICAL MECHANISMS PREVENTING GASTROESOPHAGEAL REFLUX

There are multiple physiological mechanisms that prevent the reflux of gastric contents into the distal esophagus, any alteration causes chronic esophagitis, with its consequence, intestinal metaplasia or Barrett's esophagus. These mechanisms are:

- The length of the abdominal esophagus. Thus, a key element in all antireflux surgeries is restoration of 3–4 cm of the esophagus into the abdomen (Lerut *et al.*, 2011).
- Anatomical relationship of the esophagus with the diaphragm, which compresses the esophagus, functioning as a lower esophageal sphincter.
- The oblique disposition of the cardiac orifice.
- Acute angle of His and the mucosal fold determined by the cardiac notch.
- The gastric oblique muscle distribution over the cardiac notch.

THE ANATOMICAL RELATIONSHIPS

- Anteriorly: The anterior vagal trunk, peritoneum, and the left lobe of the liver.
- Posteriorly: The posterior vagal trunk, the pillar of the diaphragm, the median arcuate ligament, the aortic hiatus of the diaphragm, and the descending aorta.
- To the right: The left lobe of liver.

The peritoneum covers the anterior and left side of the abdominal esophagus. From the right side of the esophagus, the peritoneum forms the hepatoesophageal ligament, a part of the lesser omentum.

THE VASCULAR SUPPLY

THE ARTERIES

- The left gastric artery, deriving from the celiac artery. From its convexity, is branching off the cardio-oesophageal artery for the anterior and right walls of the abdominal esophagus.

- The short gastric arteries, branching off of the splenic artery.
- The left inferior phrenic artery, which emerges from the abdominal aorta.

The periesophageal branches of the supplying arteries, enter the esophageal wall and form a rich submucosal network, that allows viability over a long distance after surgical mobilization of the organ.

The celiac artery is the first visceral branch of the abdominal aorta, immediately below the median arcuate ligament, at the level of the T12 vertebra. After a short segment of 1 cm it divides into three branches: the left gastric, the common hepatic and the splenic artery. On its sides are located the two sympathetic semilunar ganglia.

THE VEINS

The abdominal esophagus is the location of an important visceral portal-systemic anastomosis. The gastric submucosa has a venous network, close to the gastroesophageal junction it crosses the muscularis mucosa. In the mucosa, these veins form a plexus of parallel vertical lines – a "palisade zone", above the gastroesophageal junction they cross the muscularis mucosa to enrich again the submucosa. The blood from this mucosal gastroesophageal plexus drains:

- Inferiorly, through the left gastric vein into the portal vein (the preferential manner of drainage).
- Superiorly through the inferior left phrenic vein into the inferior vena cava. Ascending, through the esophageal veins, the blood drains into the hemiazygos and azygos veins, and from here into the superior vena cava.

When there is an obstacle to portal blood flow, portal hypertension, will divert the blood flow through the mucosal esophagogastric venous plexus to the superior vena cava, giving rise to esophageal varices.

THE LYMPHATICS

The lymphatic capillaries form a rich submucosal network, with longitudinal flow of the esophageal lymph. Important to note is that there is no segmental lymphatic drainage of the esophagus, any neoplasm can metastasize to the upper lymph nodes, with a frequency as high as 30% for a lower esophageal tumor.

The lymphatic flow is bidirectional, cranial and caudal, and the direction is favored by the esophageal contractility. The longitudinal course of the lymphatic capillaries into the submucosa may explain the axial spreading of cancer cells, long distances into the esophageal wall before metastasizing in the regional lymph nodes. Tracheal bifurcation represents a watershed for lymphatic drainage, with drainage into the paratracheal and cervical lymph nodes from the superior esophagus and into the lower mediastinal and celiac lymph nodes from the esophagus inferior to the bifurcation (Lerut et al., 2011).

The lymphatics of the abdominal esophagus drain to:

- The left gastric and then into the celiac lymph nodes.
- The inferior diaphragmatic lymph nodes.

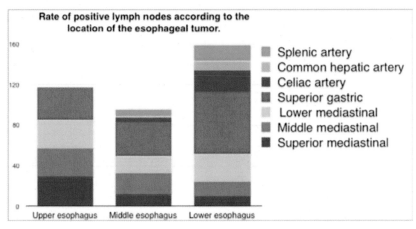

Figure 39. Rate of positive lymph nodes correlated with localization of the tumor in 210 resections for esophageal carcinoma, with extensive lymph node dissection in the posterior mediastinum and abdomen [Adapted after (Akiyama *et al.*, 1981)].

It should be noted that the direct drainage of the middle thoracic esophagus into the thoracic duct, occurs with a frequency reported by autopsy studies by as much as 43% (Broering, Walter and Halata, 2009; Lerut *et al.*, 2011).

Table 3
Lymph node stations of the esophagus (Broering, Walter and Halata, 2009;
Japan Esophageal Society, 2009; Edge *et al.*, 2010)

Lymph node(LNs) stations	Japanese classification	AJCC
Cervical LNs	100 – Superficial 101 – Paraesophageal 102 – Deep cervical 103 – Perypharyngeal 104 – Supraclavicular	1 – Supraclavicular
Thoracic LNs	105, 108, 110 – Paraesophageal 106 – Paratracheal 107 – Subcarinal 109 – Bronchopulmonary 111 – Supradiaphragmatic 112 – Posterior mediastinal	2R,2L – Right and left upper paratracheal 3P – Posterior mediastinal 4R,4L – Right and left lower paratracheal 5 – Aortopulmonary 6 – Anterior mediastinal 7 – Subcarinal nodes 8M – Middle paraesophageal 8L,8R – Lower paraesophageal 9 – Pulmonary ligament 10R,10L – Right and left tracheobronchial 15 – Diaphragmatic
Abdominal LNs	1 – Left paracardial 2 – Right paracardial 3 – Lesser curvature 4 – Greater curvature 5 – Suprapyloric 6 – Infrapyloric 7 – Left gastric	16 – Paracardial 17 – Left gastric 18 – Common hepatic 19 – Splenic 20 – Celiac

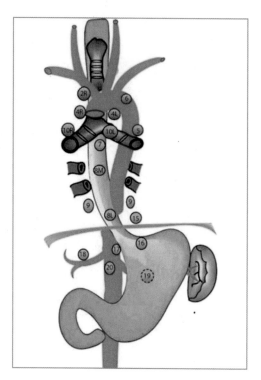

Figure 40. Schematic representation, anterior view, of the esophageal lymph node stations according to the American Joint Committee on Cancer (AJCC) [Image redrawn by IN from Simon Law (Law, 2011)].

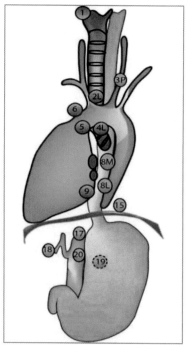

Figure 41. Schematic representation, lateral view, of the esophageal lymph node stations according to the American Joint Committee on Cancer (AJCC) [Image redrawn by IN from Simon Law (Law, 2011)].

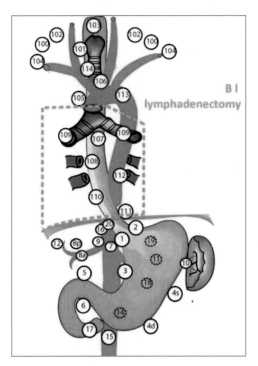

Figure 42. Schematic representation of the esophageal lymph node stations according to the Japanese Society for Esophageal Disease. The standard mediastinal lymphadenectomy (BI) is defined as an infracarinal one [Image redrawn by IN from Simon Law (Law, 2011)].

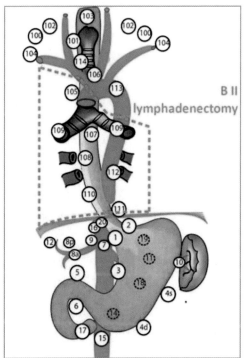

Figure 43. Schematic representation of the esophageal lymph node stations according to the Japanese Society for Esophageal Disease. The extended mediastinal lymphadenectomy (BII) is defined as BI plus upper mediastinal group along the right laryngeal recurrent nerve and right paratracheal area [Image redrawn by IN from Simon Law (Law, 2011)].

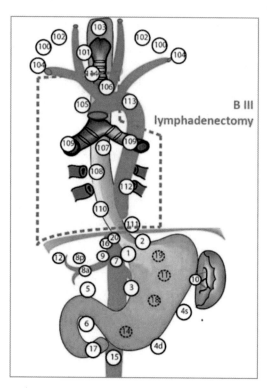

Figure 44. Schematic representation of the esophageal lymph node stations according to the Japanese Society for Esophageal Disease. The complete mediastinal lympha-denectomy (BIII) is defined as BII plus left laryngeal recurrent nerve, including the left paratracheal and subaortic areas. The three-field lymphadenecomy includes: (1) the abdominal compartment, with the celiac lymph nodes; (2) the mediastinum, with complete mediastinal clearance (BIII) and (3) bilateral cervical lymph nodes [Image redrawn by IN from Simon Law (Law, 2011)].

Table 4
Stratification of lymph nodes according to their distance
from the esophagus (Lerut *et al.*, 2011)

Level I LNs	Level II LNs	Level III LNs
Paraesophageal	Mediastinal	Lateral clavicular
	Periaortic	Pulmonary hilar
	Deep cervical	Greater curvature of the stomach
	Supraclavicular	Splenic
	Left gastric	Common hepatic
	Celiac	

Table 5

5-Year survival rate in patients with two field versus three field lymphadenectomy according to the involvement of mediastinal and abdominal lymph nodes, regardless of cervical lymph node metastasis [Adapted after (Akiyama H., Tsurumaru M., Ono Y., Udagawa H., 1991)]

Lymphnodes involvement		5-year survival	
Mediastinal	Abdominal	Thoraco-abdominal lymph node dissection	Cervical-thoraco-abdominal dissection
No	No	52.1%	75.2%
Yes	Yes	13.7%	27.4%
Yes	No	25.9%	42.7%
No	Yes	38.7%	60.2%

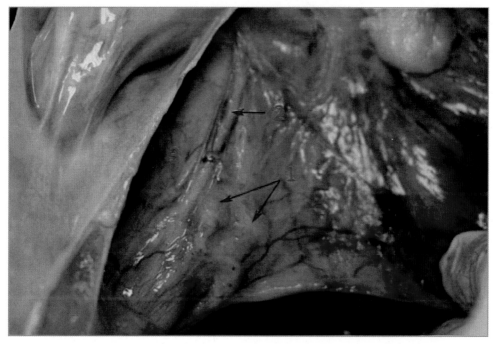

Figure 45. Dissection on a cadaveric model revealing lower paraesophageal lymph nodes (1) (station 110 according to the Japanese classification or 8L according to the AJCC staging). 2 – left vagus nerve, 3 – lower thoracic esophagus (Image personal courtesy of SH, IN).

THE NERVES

The parasympathetic innervation of the abdominal esophagus is via the two, anterior and posterior, vagal trunks.

The sympathetic fibers are from the celiac plexus. They reach the esophagus on the periarterial plexuses of the left gastric and the left inferior phrenic arteries.

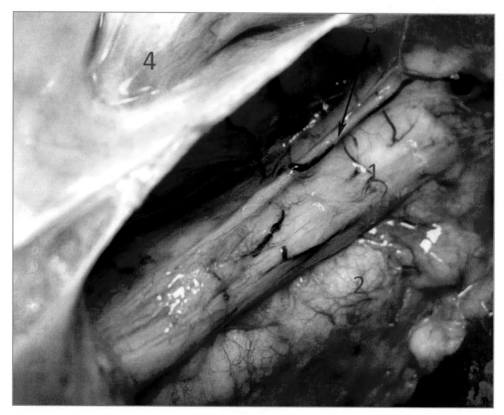

Figure 46. Dissection on a cadaveric model revealing the lower thoracic esophagus into the posterior mediastinum (1). 2 – descending thoracic aorta, 3 – left vagus nerve, 4 – inferior vena cava just below the right atrium (Image personal courtesy of SH, IN).

CHAPTER 10
HISTOLOGY

SORIN HOSTIUC, ALEXANDRU RUNCANU

The layers of the esophageal wall are:

• The mucosa – with squamous epithelium, lamina propria and muscularis mucosa.

• The submucosa – connective tissue and glands, rich longitudinal network of arterial, venous and lymphatic capillaries.

• The muscular layer – with striated muscle in the upper third, mixed striated and smooth fibers in the middle third, and smooth muscular fibers in the lower third. The muscular layer is composed of circular musculature inside and a longitudinal muscular layer outside. The longitudinal muscle layer presents an important elastic force, which makes resection of shorter esophageal segments, in trauma for example, with subsequent esophagoesophageal anastomosis almost impossible (Lerut *et al.*, 2011).

• Adventitial tissue above the diaphragm, and serosa in the abdominal esophagus.

Esophageal atresia is a congenital defect characterized by the narrowing of the esophagus. The most common variants are associated with a closed upper esophagus that connects to the windpipe instead of the lower esophagus (Spitz, Kiely and Brereton, 1987).

Esophageal diverticuli – the development of sacs or pouches from the esophagus. The most common are:

• Zenker (pharyngeal) – characterized by the posterior outpouching of the mucosal and submucosal layers through the cricopharyngeal muscle (Ellis *et al.*, 1969).

• Midesophageal (traction) – located in the middle portion of the esophagus, and mainly caused by mediastinal inflammatory lesions or esophageal motility disorders.

• Epiphrenic – usually associated with a motility disorder of the esophagus (Benacci *et al.*, 1993).

Achalasia is caused by failure of smooth muscle fiber relaxation, causing the lower esophageal sphincter to remain closed. It is associated with a chronic inflammatory response containing CD3/CD8 positive T lymphocytes, loss of ganglion cells and neurofibrosis (Clark *et al.*, 2000).

Reflux esophagitis is caused by changes in the gastric-esophageal barrier, due to hiatal hernia, obesity, Zollinger-Ellison syndrome, scleroderma, Glenard syndrome, etc. It can be transitory or definitive, and it may cause a series of complications including necrosis of the esophageal epithelium (with subsequent ulcers near the gastro-esophageal junction), esophageal strictures, Barrett's esophagus, or even esophageal adenocarcinoma (Dodds *et al.*, 1982).

Barrett's esophagus is caused by the replacement of the normal, stratified squamous epithelium in the lower esophagus with simple columnar epithelium and associated goblet cells (usually present in the lower gastrointestinal system), as a result of gastric reflux toward the esophagus. They are premalignant lesions, which can potentially lead to esophagogastric junctional adenocarcinoma (Cameron *et al.*, 1995).

Squamous cell carcinoma is usually caused by the synergic effects of tobacco and alcohol on the esophageal epithelium. It is usually located in the middle/lower part of the esophagus. Grossly, the tumor is usually circumferential, ulcerated, with sharply demarcated margins and greyish-white in color (Rosai, 2011). It has positive immunostaining for keratins, some also for vimentin or neurofilaments (Kim *et al.*, 2010). Metastases occur frequently, often in the perisesophageal area, cervical node, below the diaphragm, but also in distant organs like liver, lung or adrenal glands (Rosai, 2011).

Esophageal adenocarcinoma usually appears on columnar metaplasia (Barrett's esophagus). The tumor is usually identified in later stages, often stage IV, and subsequently the five-year survival rate is very low (around 14.5%) (Rosai, 2011).

SECTION V – THE STOMACH

*In the world of surgical oncology: Biology is King,
Selection is Queen, Technical maneuver is the Prince.*

Blake Cady

CHAPTER 11

EMBRYOLOGY

RUXANDRA IRINA NEGOI

During the fourth week of embryological development, the stomach appears as a fusiform dilation of the foregut, with a high position in the cervical region (Moore and Persaud, 2008). With the body walls growing and the development of the heart and the diaphragm, the stomach will descend into its final, abdominal position.

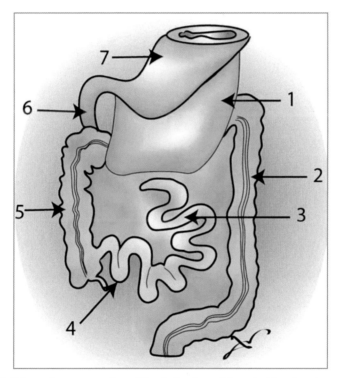

Figure 47. Schematic representation of the derivatives of the primitive dorsal mesenterium: 1 – dorsal mesogastrium, 2 – descending colon, 3 – jejunum, 4 – ileum, 5 – ascending colon, 6 – duodenum, 7 – stomach (Personal courtesy IN).

The stomach has a ventral primitive mesentery and a dorsal primitive mesentery. It has unequal growth of the margins: the anterior margin grows less and forms the lesser curvature, while the posterior margin grows more and will become the greater curvature. Starting from a sagittal disposition, the stomach will have a 90 degrees clockwise rotation (viewed from the cranial part). This rotation is due to the development of the hepatocystic bud between the layers of the ventral primitive mesentery. Secondary to this process, the lesser curvature will be located to the right and the greater curvature to the left. This rotation explains the innervation of the anterior gastric surface by the left vagus nerve and of the posterior surface by the right vagus nerve (Moore and Persaud, 2008).

The rotation of the stomach and of the duodenal loop, together with the pancreatic and hepatocystic buds, results in the appearance of the lesser peritoneal cavity or omental bursa (Negoi et al., 2010).

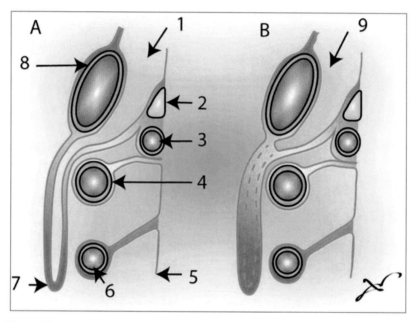

Figure 48. Schematic representation of a sagittal section through the lesser peritoneal cavity, before (A) and after (B) fusion of the primitive dorsal mesogastrium with the transverse mesocolon: 1 and 9 – omental bursa, 2 – pancreas, 3 – third duodenal segment, 4 – transverse colon, 5 – parietal peritoneum covering the retroperitoneal space, 6 – small bowel loop, 7 – folded dorsal mesogastrium, forming the gastrocolic ligament and the greater omentum (Personal courtesy IN).

After the stomach's rotation, the segment of the primitive dorsal meso-gastrium, between the gastric greater curvature and the spleen, continues to elongate and reflects over the transverse colon and mesocolon. Initially this elongation of the dorsal mesogastrium is reflected anteriorly to the transverse colon and has four peritoneal layers.

The internal ones will fuse, in adults they give rise to the greater omentum, covered by peritoneum on its anterior and posterior surfaces (two layers of peritoneum) (Sadler, 2009). The bulging of the dorsal mesogastrium is located in close proximity to the transverse mesocolon, fusing with this mesocolon. This bloodless embryological plane of fusion, between the posterior lamina of the greater omentum and the anterior lamina of the transverse mesocolon, is accessed during surgical resections for gastric and pancreatic malignancies.

Following the development of the hepatocystic bud into the ventral mesentery and of the spleen into the dorsal mesentery, around the stomach will appear the following peritoneal ligaments:

• The ventral mesentery is divided into the lesser omentum and the four peritoneal ligaments of the liver (falciform, coronary and two triangulars).

• The dorsal mesentery derivatives are the splenorenal and gastrosplenic ligaments.

CHAPTER 12

ANATOMY

MIRCEA BEURAN, IONUȚ NEGOI

The stomach is a dilated portion of the upper digestive tract, located between the esophagus and the duodenum, with a capacity in adults of about 1500 ml. A descriptive view of the stomach reveals anterior and posterior surfaces, a lesser and a greater curvature and a cardiac and a pyloric orifice.

THE PERITONEAL STRUCTURES AROUND THE STOMACH

THE LESSER OMENTUM

The lesser omentum is a peritoneal structure which connects the liver hilum with the abdominal esophagus, the lesser curvature of the stomach and the first part of the duodenum. According to its topography, the lesser omentum can be divided into three parts:

• The hepatoesophageal ligament: within which can be found the hepatic branch of the anterior vagus nerve, and in some instances an accessory left hepatic artery, branching off of the left gastric artery.

• The hepatogastric ligament: the thinnest area, consisting only of the two peritoneal lamina. Within its layers are located the hepatic branch of the left vagus nerve, and when present, an accessory or replaced left hepatic artery originating from the left gastric artery.

• The hepatoduodenal ligament: within which can be found the liver's pedicle elements, such as the portal vein, the proper hepatic artery and the common bile duct.

THE OMENTAL BURSA

The omental bursa or the lesser peritoneal cavity, is located posteriorly to the stomach, and communicates with the greater peritoneal cavity through Winslow's foramen (Negoi *et al.*, 2010). The anatomical boundaries of the Winslow orifice are:

- Anteriorly: Hepatoduodenal ligament containing the hepatic pedicle (portal vein, proper hepatic artery and common bile duct).
- Posteriorly: Inferior vena cava.
- Superiorly: Caudate lobe of liver.
- Inferiorly: First segment of the duodenum.

The anatomical boundaries of the omental bursa are:

- Anteriorly: The posterior wall of the stomach, the lesser omentum, and the gastrocolic ligament.
- Posteriorly: The anterior surface of the pancreas, the abdominal aorta, the right diaphragmatic pillar, the inferior vena cava, and the diaphragm.
- Inferiorly: The transverse colon and its mesocolon.
- Superiorly: The caudate lobe of the liver, the diaphragm, underside of the gastrophrenic ligament.

THE VASCULAR SUPPLY

THE ARTERIES

The stomach is one of the most well vascularized organs, its arterial supply accomplished by several sources, which anastomose both inside and outside the organ's wall. If at least one of its arteries are surgically preserved, the stomach will still be viable. There are five arterial sources:

- The left gastric artery, branches off of the celiac artery in the majority of cases, with 2.5–7.5% originating directly from the aorta. From its retroperitoneal origin, the artery has an ascending trajectory to the lesser curvature of the stomach. From its most superior point emerges the cardioesophageal branch. On the lesser curvature of the stomach it is divided into an anterior and a posterior branch, which anastomose with corresponding arteries from the right gastric artery. We should always remember that there is the possibility of an accessory or replaced left hepatic artery emerging from the left gastric artery, reported by Huang *et al.* with a frequency of 11.5% (Huang *et al.*, 2013).
- The right gastric artery, branches off from the proper hepatic artery.
- The left gastroepiploic artery, the largest branch of the splenic artery, branches off into the splenic hilum. It has an inferior trajectory, into the gastro-splenic and gastrocolic ligaments, parallel with the greater curvature of the stomach, 1–2 cm apart. It anastomoses in the gastrocolic ligament with the right gastroepiploic

artery. Branching off from the left and right gastroepiloic arteries are epiploic branches for the greater omentum. Two large epiploic arteries, termed the left and right epiploic arteries anastomose inside the greater omentum, forming the arc of Barkow (Lin and Chaikof, 2000). The epiploic arcade of Barkow gives off multiple small branches that communicate with the middle colic artery (Lin and Chaikof, 2000).

• The right gastroepiploic artery is one of the terminal branches of the gastroduodenal artery, together with the anterosuperior pancreaticoduodenal artery. The infrapyloric artery arises from the right gastroepiploic artery in 85% and from the gastroduodenal artery in 15% of cases.

• The short gastric arteries, are 5–7 vessels, originating from the distal splenic artery. Through the gastrosplenic ligament these vessels reach the fundus of the stomach.

• In 50–66% of patients, may be present a posterior gastric artery, with the origin in the middle segment of the splenic artery.

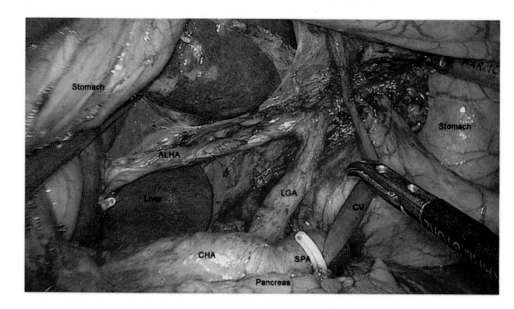

Figure 49. Intraoperative exposure of the origin and terminus of the accessory left hepatic artery (ALHA) though meticulous dissection. bLGA, left gastric artery; SPA, splenic artery; CHA, common hepatic artery; CV, coronary vein. doi:10.1371/journal.pone.0064300.g002 (Reproduced from Huang C-M, Chen Q-Y, Lin J-X, Zheng C-H, Li P, Xie J-W, *et al.* (2013) Short-Term Clinical Implications of the Accessory Left Hepatic Artery in Patients Undergoing Radical Gastrectomy for Gastric Cancer. PLoS ONE 8(5): e64300. doi:10.1371/journal.pone.0064300) (Huang *et al.*, 2013).

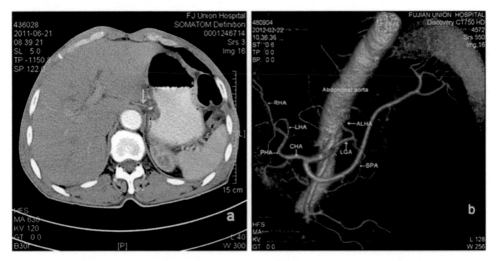

Figure 50. Preoperative enhanced transverse CT image showing a fine accessory left hepatic artery (ALHA) in the gastrohepatic ligament: (a). Three-dimensional CT reconstruction, showing an ALHA originating from the left gastric artery. (b). LGA, left gastric artery; SPA, splenic artery; CHA, common hepatic artery; PHA, proper hepatic artery; LHA, left hepatic artery; RHA, right hepatic artery. doi:10.1371/journal.pone.0064300.g003 (Reproduced from Huang C-M, Chen Q-Y, Lin J-X, Zheng C-H, Li P, Xie J-W, *et al.* (2013) Short-Term Clinical Implications of the Accessory Left Hepatic Artery in Patients Undergoing Radical Gastrectomy for Gastric Cancer. PLoS ONE 8(5): e64300. doi:10.1371/journal.pone.0064300) (Huang *et al.*, 2013).

Table 6
Adachi's classification of the celiac artery branching pattern (Huang and Zheng, 2015a)

	Frequency	Anatomical description
Type I	88.1%	CT dividing in LGA, SPA and CHA
Type II	6.3%:	LGA coming from AO CT dividing in CHA and SPA.
Type III	1.2%	LGA from AO CA dividing in CHA, SPA and SMA
Type IV	2.4%	CA dividing in LGA, CHA, SPA and SMA
Type V	0.4%	LGA and SPA coming from a common trunk, with origin in AO CHA and SMA common origin in CA
Type VI	2%	LGA and SPA from CA CHA issues from the SMA

CA – celiac artery, LGA – left gastric artery, CHA – common hepatic artery, SPA – splenic artery, AO – aorta, SMA – superior mesenteric artery.

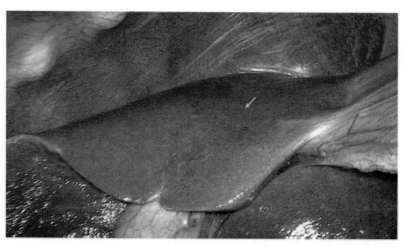

Figure 51. Image showing impairment of the blood supply to the left hepatic parenchyma after a relatively large accessory left hepatic artery (ALHA) was severed (arrows). doi:10.1371/journal.pone.0064300.g004 (Reproduced from Huang C-M, Chen Q-Y, Lin J-X, Zheng C-H, Li P, Xie J-W, *et al.* (2013) Short-Term Clinical Implications of the Accessory Left Hepatic Artery in Patients Undergoing Radical Gastrectomy for Gastric Cancer. PLoS ONE 8(5): e64300. doi:10.1371/journal. pone.0064300) (Huang *et al.*, 2013).

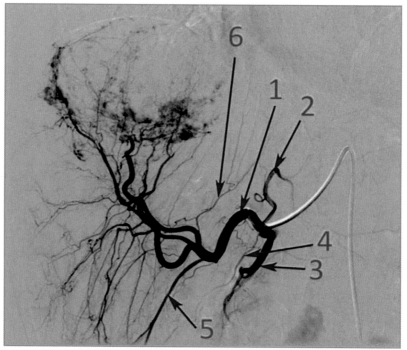

Figure 52. Angiography of the celiac artery revealing the common hepatic artery (1), left gastric artery (2), splenic artery (3), dorsal pancreatic artery (4), gastroduodenal artery (5) and left hepatic artery (6) (Figure courtesy of Emergency Hospital of Bucharest, Department of Angiography).

THE VEINS

The venous return of the stomach drains into the portal vein. The left gastric vein drains into the portal vein trunk or into the splenic vein. The area near the left gastric vein is challenging to dissect during lymphadenectomy for cancer. The left gastric vein is small and fragile, and can be easily torn during suprapancreatic lymph node dissection in patients with pancreatic cancer (Lin JX, 2013). The introduction of multidetector computed tomography to assess the perigastric vascular anatomy during preoperative planning is associated with significantly less intraoperative blood loss (158.6 ml *versus* 94.1 ml, p = 0.0032) (Miyaki *et al.*, 2012).

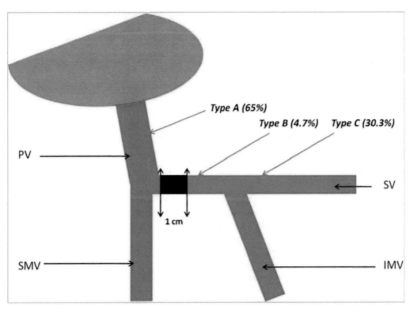

Figure 53. Left gastric vein (LGV) termination sites and their frequencies. Type a: termination on the portal vein (PV); Type b: termination on the spleno-mesenteric trunk (SMT); Type c: termination on the splenic vein (SV); SMV: superior mesenteric vein; IMV: inferior mesenteric vein. The distance between the termination of the LGV (when located on the SMT or the SV) and the origin of the PV was always greater than 10 mm (the zone delimited by the black box) [Figure reproduced with permission from John Wiley and Sons from Lionel Rebibo,Cyril Chivot, David Fuks, Charles Sabbagh, Thierry Yzet, Jean-Marc Regimbeau. Three-dimensional computed tomography analysis of the left gastric vein in a pancreatectomy. HPB – The Official Journal of the International Hepato Pancreato Biliary Association. 14 (6), 414–421, 2012 (Rebibo *et al.*, 2012)].

Its preoperative localization is important, with a sensitivity for CT of 93.8% (Kawasaki *et al.*, 2010). In their study, Kawasaki *et al.* found a left gastric vein located dorsal to the common hepatic artery in 49.4%, ventral to the common hepatic artery in 22.2%, ventral to the splenic artery in 21%, dorsal to the splenic artery in 2.5% and in other positions in 4.9% (Kawasaki *et al.*, 2010). Natsume *et al.* evaluated the anatomic variations of the left gastric vein in 126 consecutive patients (92 – gastric cancer, 10 – gastric GIST, 7 – colorectal cancer and 17 others), using a 64-row CT (Natsume *et al.*, 2010). They found that the left gastric vein ran posterior to the common hepatic artery in 39.2% and in 22.4% it ran anterior to the splenic artery (Natsume *et al.*, 2010). In two out of 245 Japanese cadavers, Miyaki *et al.* found a left hepatic vein entering the left side of the hepatogastric ligament from the cardiac region, running towards the left side of the hepatic hilum and joining the intrahepatic ramification of the portal vein (Miyaki, Yamada and Kumaki, 1987). This configuration, with an aberrant left gastric vein draining directly into the liver may correspond to the phylogenetic and ontogenetic "left portal vein" (Ohkubo, 2000). In their analyses of 2111 patients, Huang *et al.* found a mean diameter of the left gastric vein of 5.10 ± 0.40 mm, a mean length of 37.40 ± 5.19 mm, and a mean distance between the end of the left gastric vein and the splenoportal confluence of 13.05 ± 0.86 mm (Huang *et al.*, 2014a).

The right gastric vein has a mean diameter of 2.18 mm. It receives the prepyloric vein of Mayo, which presents a vertical subserosal trajectory, anterior to the pyloric sphincter.

The left gastroepiploic vein drains into the splenic vein. The right gastroepiploic vein joins the anterosuperior pancreaticoduodenal vein and an accessory right colic vein, forming the gastrocolic trunk of Henle. This drains into the superior mesenteric vein.

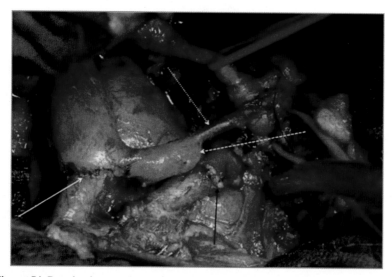

Figure 54. Portal vein resection and resection of the splenic vein with preservation of the coronary vein (anatomical situation type 2). White arrow: portal vein anastomosis; dotted white arrow: coronary vein; broken white arrow: splenic vein; black arrow: additional superior mesenteric artery anastomosis [Figure reproduced with permission from John Wiley and Sons from Thilo Hackert, Jürgen Weitz, Markus W. Büchler. Reinsertion of the gastric coronary vein to avoid venous gastric congestion in pancreatic surgery. HPB, 17 (4), 368–370, 2015, (Hackert, Weitz and Büchler, 2015)].

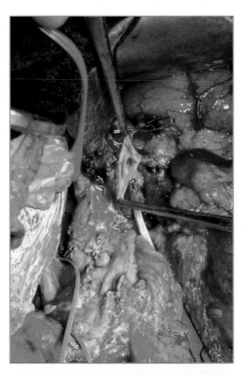

Figure 55. Mobilization and preparation of the coronary vein. A patch of the splenic vein is preserved for the anastomosis (between the forceps). Intraoperative venous congestion of the stomach is visible (right upper corner) [Figure reproduced with permission from John Wiley and Sons from Thilo Hackert, Jürgen Weitz, Markus W. Büchler. Reinsertion of the gastric coronary vein to avoid venous gastric congestion in pancreatic surgery. HPB, 17 (4), 368–370, 2015, (Hackert, Weitz and Büchler, 2015)].

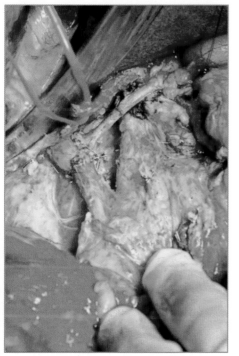

Figure 56. Completed anastomosis of the coronary vein. The vein is re-inserted above the portal vein anastomosis created previously. Restoration of the stomach drainage can be seen by release of the venous congestion (right upper corner) [Figure reproduced with permission from John Wiley and Sons from Thilo Hackert, Jürgen Weitz, Markus W. Büchler. Reinsertion of the gastric coronary vein to avoid venous gastric congestion in pancreatic surgery. HPB, 17 (4), 368–370, 2015, (Hackert, Weitz and Büchler, 2015)].

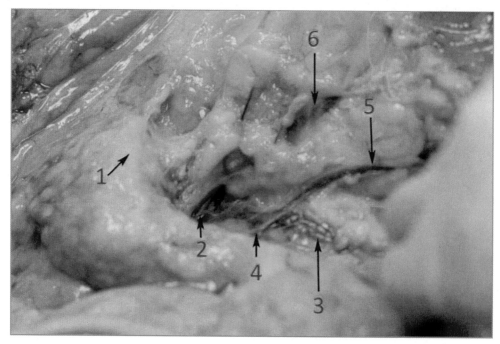

Figure 57. Dissection on a cadaveric model. Can be observed, the inferior margin of the pancreas (1), Henle's trunk draining into the superior mesenteric vein (2), the right gastroepiploic vein (3), anterior superior pancreaticoduodenal vein (4), right superior colic vein (5) and middle colic vein (6) (Image courtesy of SH, IN).

THE LYMPHATICS

The stomach has a rich lymphatic network. Studies on lymph drainage pathways in gastric cancer revealed that metastasis can "jump" to higher lymph node stations, rather than invading the closest nodes, followed by continuous spreading (Choi *et al.*, 2015; Kim *et al.*, 2015).

Table 7
Lymph node stations according to the Japanese Society (Japan Esophageal Society, 2009; Japanese Gastric Cancer Association, 2011; Huang and Zheng, 2015b)

Group No.	Anatomical location
1	Right cardiac – along the ascending branch of the left gastric artery, located on the anterior and right sides of the cardia.
2	Left cardiac – along the esophagogastric branch of the left inferior phrenic artery, located on the left and posterior sides of the cardia.
3	Lesser curvature – into the lesser omentum.
4	Greater curvature: 4sa – along short gastric vessels. 4sb – along left gastroepiploic vessels, starting with the first gastric branch. 4d – along the right gastroepiploic vessels, starting with the second branch.

Table 7 (continous)

5	Suprapyloric – along the proximal part and first branch of the right gastric artery.
6	Infrapyloric – along the proximal part of the right gastroepiploic artery and its first branch, down to the confluence of the right gastroepiploic vein with the anterosuperior pancreaticoduodenal vein.
7	Left gastric – around the left gastric artery, starting with its origin and up to the ascending branch.
8	Common hepatic : 8a – anterosuperior group, from the origin of the common hepatic until the emergence of the gastroduodenal artery. 8p – posterior group, which are continuous with 12p and 16a2.
9	Celiac artery, around the celiac trunk.
10	Splenic hilum, around the splenic artery, distal to the pancreatic tail, around the root of the short gastric and around the left gastroepiploic artery before its first gastric branch.
11	Splenic artery: 11p – along the proximal splenic artery, between the origin and the midpoint origin – pancreatic tail. 11d – along the distal splenic artery, midpoint origin – pancreatic tail to the end of the pancreatic tail.
12	Hepatoduodenal ligament : 12a – along the proper hepatic artery, below the confluence of the right and left hepatic ducts and above the pancreatic border. 12b – along the bile duct 12p – along the portal vein
13	Posterior surface of the pancreatic head
14	Along the superior mesenteric vessels: 14a – along the superior mesenteric artery 14v – along the superior mesenteric vein, in front of the vein, in the space with the following boundaries: <ul><li>Superiorly: inferior margin of the pancreas</li><li>Inferiorly: emergence of the middle colic vein</li><li>Right: confluence of the right gastroepiploic vein with anterosuperior pancreatico-duodenal vein.</li><li>Left: left margin of the superior mesenteric vein.</li></ul>
15	Middle colic artery
16	Around the abdominal aorta: 16a1 – in the aortic hiatus, between the diaphragmatic crura. 16a2 – around the abdominal aorta, from the upper margin of the celiac artery to the lower margin of the left renal vein 16b1 – around the abdominal aorta from the lower margin of the left renal vein to the upper margin of the inferior mesenteric artery 16b2 – around the abdominal aorta, from the upper margin of the inferior mesenteric artery to the aortic bifurcation
17	Anterior surface of the pancreatic head
18	Along the inferior margin of the pancreas
19	Infradiaphragmatic
20	In the esophageal hiatus of the diaphragm

THE NERVES

The stomach has both, parasympathetic and sympathetic autonomous innervation. The parasympathetic innervation is through both the anterior and the posterior vagal nerves. The anterior vagal nerve has gastric and liver branches. For the stomach there are 4–10 branches, descending on its anterior surface. One of these branches, a larger one, is a continuation of the anterior vagal nerve on the lesser curvature of the stomach, and is termed the main anterior nerve of the lesser curvature of Latarjet (Negoi *et al.*, 2010). The liver branch has its trajectory through the lesser omentum to the hepatic hilum, dividing there into an ascending and a descending branch. The descending fibers innervate the upper duodenum, while the ascending branches innervate the intrahepatic bile ducts and vessels. The posterior vagal nerve has gastric and celiac branches. There are 1–15 gastric branches, the larger being called the main posterior nerve of the lesser curvature of Latarjet. The celiac branches count for half of the posterior vagal nerve fibers, and reach the two celiac ganglia, bringing parasympathetic fibers to the celiac plexus. The sympathetic innervation of the stomach is formed from the postsynaptic fibers of the celiac plexus, which reach the stomach through the periarterial plexuses. The presynaptic fibers for the celiac plexus are formed from the splanchnic nerves.

CHAPTER 13

HISTOLOGY

VALENTIN ENACHE, SORIN HOSTIUC, BOGDAN STOICA

The stomach has an endocrine, an exocrine, and a digestive function. The mucosa of the stomach has a cylindrical epithelial lining, a lamina propria, and a muscularis mucosa. The submucosa consists of dense connective tissue, including the Meissner plexus, blood and lymph vessels. The muscular layer presents an inner layer of oblique fibers, a middle layer of circular fibers and an external layer of longitudinal fibers. Inside this muscular layer is located the myenteric plexus of Auerbach. The external layer of the stomach is represented by the peritoneum.

Acute gastritis is characterized as an acute mucosal inflammatory reaction, and includes acute hemorrhage and acute erosive gastritis. Initially it produces edema of the lamina propria, vascular congestion, scattered foci of hemorrhage and neutrophils. If the inflammatory process is more severe, a loss of the superficial epithelium, hemorrhage, acute inflammatory infiltrate, puss, and regenerative changes of the nearby epithelium are identifiable (Brown, Davidson and Larson, 1989; Rocha *et al.*, 1991).

Chronic gastritis is characterized by the presence of a chronic inflammatory infiltration in the lamina propria which is associated with atrophy of the glandular epithelium. The main causes are Helicobacter pylori, and the use of NSAIDS, but it may appear in association with Crohn's disease, liver or kidney failure, or various connective tissue disorders (Whitehead, Truelove and Gear, 1972; Correa, 1988; Yao, 2014).

Peptic ulcers are characterized by a loss of substance involving more than just the superficial gastric layers. They are usually located on the lesser gastric curvature or on the duodenum (Lundell, Vieth and Gibson, 2015). Grossly, they are identifiable through a round/ovoid loss of substance, with slightly elevated borders and a finely granular base. During its active phase, it presents four areas: inflammatory exudate, fibrin necrosis, granulation tissue and fibrous tissue. It may lead to upper gastrointestinal bleeding, perforation, penetration, peritonitis, gastric stenosis or cancer (Lim *et al.*, 2015).

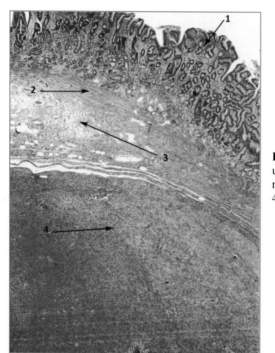

Figure 58. Hematoxylin and Eosin staining using 2.5 × objective of a gastric GIST: 1 – gastric mucosa, 2 – muscularis mucosa, 3 – submucosa, 4 – GIST (Image courtesy of VE, used with permission).

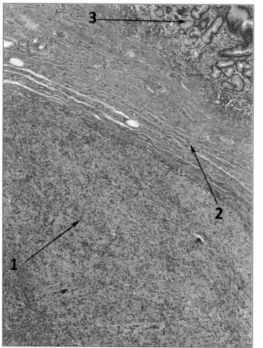

Figure 59. Hematoxylin and Eosin staining using 50 × objective of a gastric GIST: 1 – GIST, 2 – submucosa, 3 – gastric mucosa (Image courtesy of VE, used with permission).

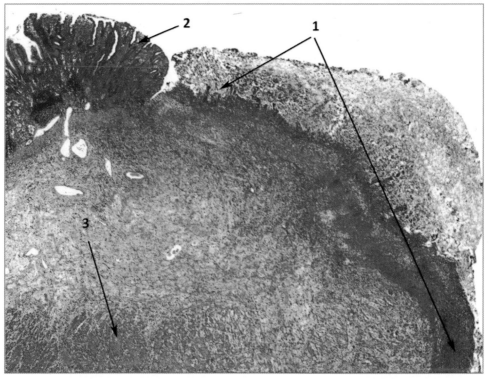

Figure 60. Hematoxylin and Eosin staining using 25 × objective of a gastric ulcer (1). Can be observed ulceration of the mucosa and submucosa, up to the muscularis propria (3). 2 – gastric mucosa with chronic inflammation (Image courtesy of VE, used with permission).

Ménétrier's disease (hypoproteinemic hypertrophic gastropathy) is characterized by the presence of massive gastric folds (mostly in the fundus and body areas) that are associated with increased mucous secretion and subsequent protein loss, caused by an increased secretion of TGFalpha (Yang *et al.*, 2015). Histologically it is characterized by the presence of massive foveolar hyperplasia, elongated glands, and cystic dilation (Lambrecht, 2011; Endo *et al.*, 2012).

Zollinger-Ellison syndrome is characterized by an increased gastric acid secretion, determined by autologous gastrin secretion from a gastrinoma, causing peptic ulcer. Grossly, are identifiable signs of reflux esophagitis, thickened gastric folds, mosaic pattern of the mucosal layer, bulbar erosions and ulcerations, and the presence of a gastrinoma (Tang, Wu and Bhaijee, 2014).

CHAPTER 14
GASTRIC CANCER

IONUȚ NEGOI, MIRCEA BEURAN

For patients with gastric cancer, the principal surgical resection with curative intent is represented by standard gastrectomy, which involves resection of at least two-thirds of the stomach with a D2 lymph node dissection (Japanese Gastric Cancer Association, 2011).

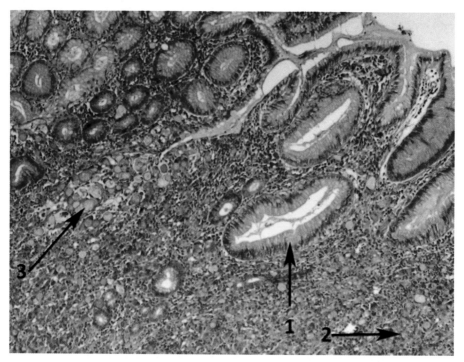

Figure 61. Hematoxylin and Eosin staining using 100 × objective of gastric diffuse adenocarcinoma (2): 1 – gastric foveola, 3 – signet ring cell adenocarcinoma (Image courtesy of VE, used with permission).

The resection margin should be at least 3 cm in expansive growth pattern tumors and of at least 5 cm in infiltrative tumors. For tumors which invade the esophagus, the 5 cm rule is not necessary, but the proximal resection line should be verified by frozen section analysis (Japanese Gastric Cancer Association, 2011). Oh *et al.* investigated the effects of spleen-preserving lymphadenectomy on surgical outcomes of locally advanced proximal gastric cancer (Oh *et al.*, 2009). Analyses of 366 patients revealed that the spleen-preservation group experienced a shorter operation time, a lower incidence of perioperative transfusion, and a shorter postoperative hospital stay. Multivariate analyses showed that tumor size, serosal invasion and nodal metastasis were independent prognostic factors, while splenectomy was not. The cumulative survival rate in pN0 patients was significantly higher in the spleen-preserving group, with no differences for pN1 and pN2 patients (Oh *et al.*, 2009). Schwartz proved the technical feasibility of spleen-preserving splenic hilar lymphadenectomy during gastrectomy for cancer (Schwarz, 2002). After distal gastrectomy, the favored reconstruction should be the Roux-en-Y. Compared to Bilroth II, the Bilroth I reconstruction is associated with a higher incidence of local recurrence rate, which may be explained by a too limited gastric resection and lymph node dissection for a tension-free anastomosis (Stange and Weitz, 2015). As the Roux-en-Y reconstruction is associated with better symptomatology related to bilio-pancreatic reflux when compared to Bilroth II reconstruction, it should be the preferred technique. After total gastrectomy, the medical evidence proved that adding a pouch to a Roux-en-Y reconstruction comes with better clinical outcomes for patients (reflux, dumping syndrome, eating capability, quality of life), at least for the first year postoperatively, without adding supplementary mortality and morbidity (Stange and Weitz, 2015).

Table 8

Type of lymphadenectomy correlated with the gastric resection according to the Japanese Gastric Cancer Association [Adapted after (Japanese Gastric Cancer Association, 2011)]

Type of gastrectomy	Lymphnodes dissection	Indications for lymphadenectomy
Total gastrectomy	D0: Less than D1 D1: Stations 1 – 7. D1+: D1 + 8a, 9, 11p D2: D1 + 8a, 9, 10, 11p, 11d, 12a Tumor invading esophagus: D1+: includes station 110 D2: includes stations 19, 20, 110, 111	D1 or D1+ for T1N0 tumors D2 for T2-T4 or N+ tumors
Distal gastrectomy	D0: Less than D1 D1: Stations 1, 3, 4sb, 4d, 5, 6, 7 D1+: D1 + 8a, 9. D2: D1+ 8a, 9, 11p, 12a.	

Table 9
Randomized controlled studies evaluating lymph node dissection in patients with gastric cancer

Study	Location/ No pts.	Outcomes	Morbidity	Mortality	Overall survival
(Bonenkamp et al., 1995; Hartgrink et al., 2004; Songun et al., 2010)	Dutch/711	D1 vs. D2	25 vs. 43% (p<0.001)	4 vs. 10% (p=0.004)	At 15 years - 21 vs. 29% (p=0.34) Gastric Cancer specific death – 48 vs. 37% (p=0.01)
(Cuschieri et al., 1996, 1999)	UK/400	D1 vs. D2	28 vs. 46% (p<0.001)	6.5 vs. 13% (p=0.04)	At 5 years – 35 vs. 33% (p=ns)
(Degiuli, Sasako and Ponti, 2010; Degiuli et al., 2014)	Italy/267	D1 vs. D2	12 vs. 17.9% (p=0.17)	3 vs. 2.2 % (p=0,72)	At 5 years: 66.5 vs. 64.2% (p=0.69)
(Sano et al., 2004; Sasako et al., 2008)	Japan/523	D2 vs. D2+	20.9 vs. 28.1% (p=0.06)	0.8 vs. 0.8%	At 5 years: 69.2 vs. 70.3% (p=0.85)
(Wu et al., 2004)	Taiwan/221	D1 vs. D3	7.3 vs. 17.1%	0 vs. 0%	At 5 years: 53.6 vs. 59.5%, (p=0.04)

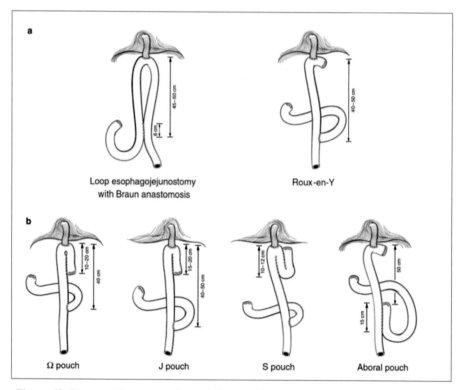

Figure 62. Roux-en-Y reconstruction techniques without a pouch (a), *versus* with pouch (b)
(Reprinted by permission from Macmillan Publishers Ltd: The American Journal of
Gastroenterology (Gertler *et al.*, 2009), copyright 2009).

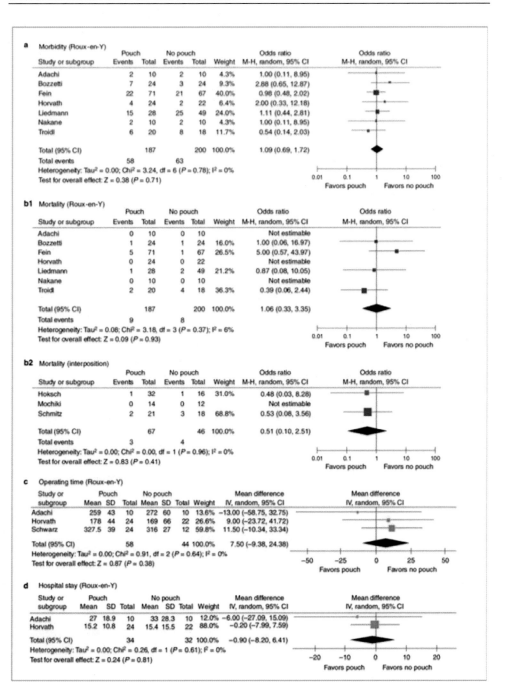

Figure 63. Meta-analyses on parameters of the postoperative course. (a) Morbidity (Roux-en-Y); (b1) mortality (Roux-en-Y); (b) mortality (interposition); (c) operating time (Roux-en-Y); (d) hospital stay (Roux-en-Y) (Reprinted by permission from Macmillan Publishers Ltd: The American Journal of Gastroenterology (Gertler et al., 2009), copyright 2009).

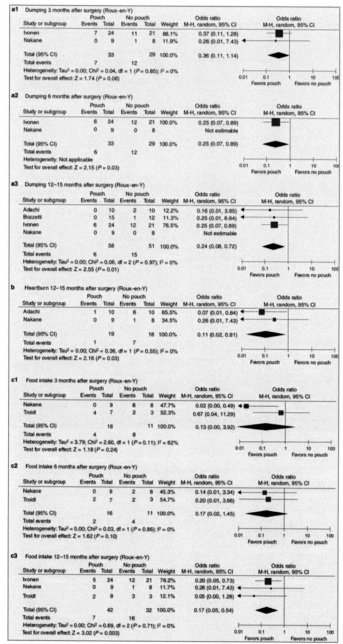

Figure 64. Meta-analyses on postgastrectomy symptoms. (a1) Dumping 3 months after surgery (Roux-en-Y); (a2) dumping 6 months after surgery (Roux-en-Y); (a3) dumping 12–15 months after surgery (Roux -en- Y); (b) heartburn 12–15 months after surgery (Roux-en-Y); (c1) food intake 3 months after surgery (Roux-en-Y); (c2) food intake 6 months after surgery (Roux-en-Y); (c3) food intake 12–15 months after surgery (Roux-en-Y) (Reprinted by permission from Macmillan Publishers Ltd: The American Journal of Gastroenterology (Gertler *et al.*, 2009), copyright 2009).

SECTION VI – THE LIVER

Everything we hear is an opinion, not a fact.
Everything we see is a perspective, not a truth.

Marcus Aurelius

CHAPTER 15

EMBRYOLOGY

RUXANDRA IRINA NEGOI

The embryological development of the liver and biliary tract starts with the hepatocystic bud, during the fourth week of intrauterine life (Moore and Persaud, 2008). The hepatocystic bud has an endodermal origin, emerging from the primitive gut, at the boundary between the foregut and the midgut. Located in the primitive ventral mesentery, the hepatocystic bud has the following segments:

The liver bud, which gives rise to the hepatocytes, and the mucosa of the intrahepatic biliary ducts, the right, left, and common hepatic ducts.

The cystic bud, which gives rise to the mucosa of the cystic duct and the gallbladder.

The common distal part of the liver and cystic buds develop into the common hepatic duct mucosa.

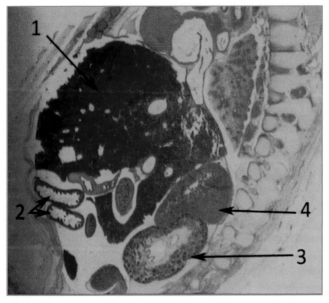

Figure 65. Sagittal section through the abdomen of a rat embryo revealing the liver (1), small bowel loops (2), kidney (3) and adrenal gland (4) (Figure personal courtesy of RIN).

The other layers of the biliary ducts have their embryological origin in the local mesenchyme (Negoi *et al.*, 2010). Just inferior to the hepatocystic bud is the origin of the ventral pancreatic bud.

During its development, the liver bud penetrates the septum transversum. The mesodermal cells of the transverse septum, interact with the endodermal cells of the liver bud which gives rise to:

The fibrous capsule of the liver, termed Glisson's capsule.

The intrahepatic connective tissue.

The hematopoietic and Kupffer cells.

Continuing its development, the liver bud interacts with the vitelline and umbilical veins, which gives rise to the hepatic sinusoids (Sadler, 2009).

The close relationship between the liver bud and the septum transversum is reflected by their direct contact in the bare area of the liver. In this area the peritoneal reflections will form the coronary and triangular ligaments.

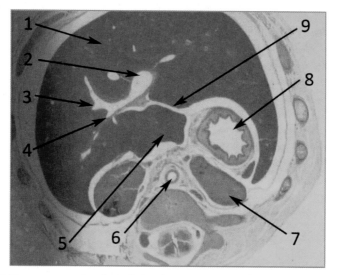

Figure 66. Transverse section through the abdomen of a rat embryo revealing the liver (1) with the left branch of the portal vein (2), right anterior (3) and posterior (4) sectional portal vein branches, caudate lobe (5), ligamentum venosum of Arantius (9). 6 – aorta, 7 – adrenal gland, 8 – stomach (Figure courtesy of RIN).

CHAPTER 16

ANATOMY

IONUȚ NEGOI, MIRCEA BEURAN

The liver is the largest parenchymal organ in the body, accounting for approximately 2%–5% of the average body weight, with a transverse diameter of 20–23 cm, and an anteroposterior diameter at the level of the right kidney of 10–12.5 cm (Negoi *et al.*, 2010). Successful liver surgery is based on (a) resection of all pathological tissue; (b) preservation of the maximum amount of healthy, well vascularized, liver parenchyma; (c) minimization of intraoperative blood loss (Poston and Blumgart, 2003).

LIVER PROJECTION ON THE THORACO-ABDOMINAL WALL

Upper boundary: the horizontal line through the fifth rib on the right mid-clavicular line and the fifth intercostal space on the left midclavicular line.

Lateral boundary: midaxillary line, from the fifth rib to the point located 2 cm inferior to the costal margin.

Lower boundary: the oblique line through the right costal margin (X^{th} rib) and the left VIIth rib's cartilage.

EXTERNAL CONFIGURATION

The liver has both a diaphragmatic and a visceral surface, and an inferior border. The diaphragmatic surface is smooth and convex, the majority of this surface is covered by visceral peritoneum. On the posterior aspect of the diaphragmatic surface, between the layers of the coronary ligament, an extraperitoneal area can be observed, termed the bare area. In this area, the liver has direct contact with the diaphragm, without interposition of the peritoneum. The posterior relationships of the liver include: the inferior vena cava, the diaphragm, the pleural recess, and the base of the right lung. The superior relationships are with the diaphragm, and through this with the right lung, the heart and pericardium. The visceral surface presents three fissures, two sagittal and one transverse. The right sagittal sulcus includes, anteriorly the gallbladder fossa and posteriorly the groove of the inferior vena cava. The left sagittal sulcus is determined, anteriorly by the round ligament and posteriorly by the venous ligament of Arantii. The transverse sulcus is determined by the liver hilum or the porta hepatica. The left lobe has posterior relationships with the abdominal esophagus and with the lesser curvature of the stomach. The right lobe has direct relationships, without interposition of the peritoneum, with the right kidney and the right adrenal gland. The right adrenal vein drains directly into the inferior vena cava, its avulsion during right hemiliver mobilization causes significant bleeding. The right hemiliver has inferior anatomical relationships with the right angle of the colon, and the first duodenal segment.

THE PERITONEUM OF THE LIVER

The liver is covered by peritoneum on most of its surface, its reflection on the abdominal wall and the neighboring structures determines the ligaments of the liver.

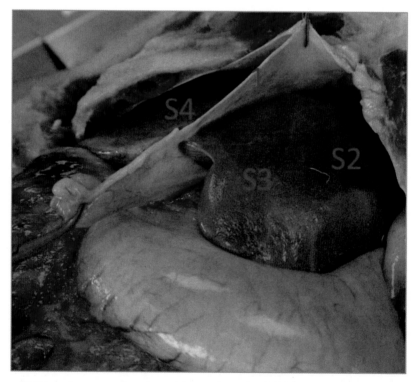

Figure 67. Dissection on a cadaveric model, revealing the falciform (1) and round (2) ligaments: S2, S3, S4 – liver segments (Image personal courtesy of SH, IN).

The lesser omentum, with its two segments, the hepatoduodenal and hepato-gastric ligaments, connects the hilum of the liver and the ligamentum venosum of Arantius fissure with the duodenum and the lesser curvature of the stomach. The hepatoduodenal ligament contains the portal vein, the proper hepatic artery and the common bile duct. During hepatic resection, at this level, complete control of the liver vascular inflow may be accomplished by a Pringle maneuver. This maneuver was developed by the Australian surgeon James Hogarth Pringle, while in Glasgow, Scotland, while managing a liver trauma (Abdel-Misih and Bloomston, 2010). The Pringle maneuver may be realized by using a vascular clamp, or less traumatically with a tourniquet.

The falciform ligament is a triangular structure, connecting the diaphragmatic surface of the liver with the anterior abdominal wall. Its inferior border contains the round ligament of the liver. At the base of the falciform ligament, along the liver may be found hepatic veins that drain into the inferior vena cava (Abdel-Misih and Bloomston, 2010).

The round ligament appears through the obliteration of the umbilical vein. The umbilical vein carries placental blood to the fetus, and starts its obliteration from the VIIth month of intrauterine life and continues during the first 2–3 years after birth. The end segment of the round ligament joins the left branch of the portal vein. The intrahepatic segment of the umbilical vein connects the left branch of the portal vein with the left hepatic vein, and will become, in adult life, the ligamentum venosum of Arantius. The ligamentum venosum is located in a fissure on the inferior surface of the liver, between the caudate lobe posteriorly and the left lobe anteriorly, and is surrounded by the peritoneum of the lesser omentum (Abdel-Misih and Bloomston, 2010).

Studying the anatomy of the ligamentum venosum in 50 human cadavers, Dahmane et al. found that it had a length of 52–70 mm and a thickness of 5–8 mm (Dahmane et al., 2009). They also found that this ligamentum had a fibrotic structure and was not patent in 96% of cases. The extrahepatic segment of the left hepatic vein measured 3–19 mm, of the middle hepatic vein 3–18 mm, and of the common trunk of the two veins 4–15 mm. The authors concluded that surgical dissection of the ligamentum venosum can facilitate extraparenchymatous clamping of the hepatic veins (Dahmane et al., 2009).

Anatomical examination of 50 livers from embalmed adults revealed that the ligamentum venosum originated from a point between the transverse and umbilical portions of the left portal vein in all specimens, and terminated in the common trunk of the middle hepatic vein and left hepatic vein in 61% of cases and in the left hepatic vein in 39% of cases (Hur, Kim and Lee, 2015). The ligamentum venosum is an anatomical landmark between the medial and lateral portions of the left portal vein. Sareli et al. found that in 8–12 % of cases the anterior sectional vein or the right-sided bile ducts transposed into the medial portion of the left portal pedicle (Sareli et al., 2009). Based on this anatomical study, the authors concluded that ligation of the left portal pedicle at its convergence with the ligamentum venosum may prevent erroneous injury of the transposed right-sided vessels or bile ducts (Sareli *et al.*, 2009). The ligamentum venosum may be patent at its cranial end, producing significant hemorrhage when a lesser omentectomy-omental bursectomy for peritoneal carcinomatosis is performed. According to this, Paul Sugarbaker recommends ligation of this anatomical structure prior to removal of the specimen from the superior aspect of the omental bursa (Sugarbaker, 2015).

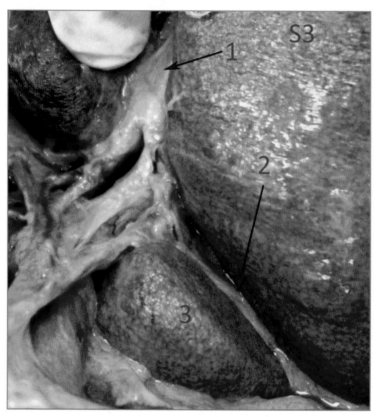

Figure 68. Dissection on a cadaveric model revealing the umbilical fissure (1), the fissure of the venous ligament of Arantius (2), the Spigelian lobe from S1 (3), S2 and S3 – liver segments (Image personal courtesy of SH, IN).

Within the falciform ligament may be found the paraumbilical veins of Sappey, which starts from the liver and ends in the periumbilical area of the abdominal wall (Skandalakis *et al.*, 2004).

The coronary ligament is determined by the posterior reflection of the peritoneum on the diaphragm. Between its superior and inferior layers is delimited the bare area of the liver. The two laminae of the coronary ligament join laterally, determining the right and left triangular ligaments. During liver surgery, to obtain adequate mobilization of the liver, all these avascular structures should be divided.

THE PORTAL VEIN

The origin of the portal vein is found posterior to the pancreatic head. Then, it has an ascending trajectory, posterior to the first segment of the duodenum, with the common bile duct being immediately anterior and to the right and the gastroduodenal artery anterior and to the left. In the hepatoduodenal ligament, the portal vein is one of the three elements of the hepatic pedicle, together with the proper hepatic artery, located anterior and to the left and the common bile duct, which is located anterior and to the right.

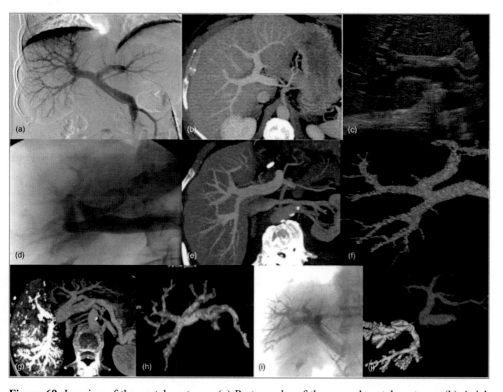

Figure 69. Imaging of the portal anatomy: (a) Portography of the normal portal anatomy. (b) Axial enhanced computed tomography (CT) scan at the portal phase of the normal portal anatomy. (c) Ultrasound (US) of normal portal anatomy. (d) Portography of type 1 portal anatomy. (e) Axial enhanced CT scan at the portal phase of type 1 portal anatomy. (f) Axial 3-D reconstruction of type 1 portal anatomy. (g) Axial enhanced CT scan of type 2 portal anatomy. (h) Axial 3-D reconstruction of type 2 portal anatomy. (i) Portography, axial 3-D reconstruction of type 3 portal anatomy. (j) Axial 3-D reconstruction of type 3 portal anatomy (Figure reproduced with permission from John Wiley and Sons from Charlotte Mouly, David Fuks, François Browet, François Mauvais, Arnaud Potier, Thierry Yzet, Qassemyar Quentin, Jean-Marc Regimbeau. Feasibility of the Glissonian approach during right hepatectomy. HPB – The Official Journal of the International Hepato Pancreato Biliary Association. 2013 15 (8), 638–645) (Mouly *et al.*, 2013).

INTRAHEPATIC DISTRIBUTION OF THE PORTAL VEIN

In the right margin of the liver hilum, the main portal vein branches off into its two main branches, the right and left. The most common variation of portal vein division is the absence of the right portal vein, the anterior and posterior sectional branches emerge directly with the left portal vein from the main portal trunk. From its origin, the right portal vein has an extrahepatic course of 1–1.5 cm.

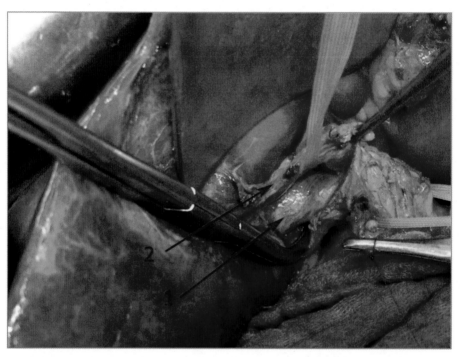

Figure 70. Intraoperative view of the right portal vein (1) and right hepatic artery (2). It should be noted that the main portal vein bifurcates into the right extremity of the liver hilum, thus the emergence of the left portal vein is very close to the area of dissection (Image from personal collection of IN).

Inside the liver parenchyma, after a very short trajectory the right portal vein divides into anterior and posterior branches, for the corresponding sections of the right hemiliver. Each of these anterior and posterior branches further divide into an ascending and descending branch, for the corresponding segments of the liver. From the initial segment of the right portal vein emerges a thin branch, for the caudate lobe. The intrahepatic distribution of the right portal vein is similar to that of the right hepatic artery and the right biliary duct.

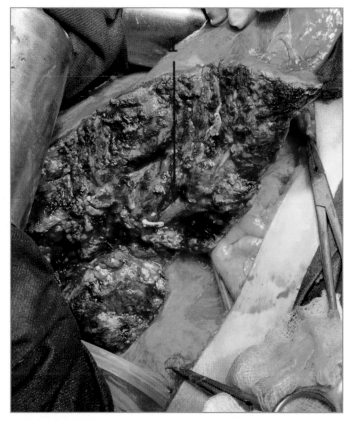

Figure 71. Intraoperative view of the transected surface of the remnant liver after resection of segments 6, 7, 8 for metachronous metastases from rectal cancer, revealing the glissonian pedicle for segment 5 (1) (Image from personal collection of IN).

The left portal vein is thinner and longer. Initially, it has a transverse or horizontal portion, of 3–4 cm, from the right to left margin of the liver hilum, at the base of segment 4. This initial transverse segment of the left portal vein is separated from the undersurface of segment 4 by connective tissue, termed the hilar plate (Hann, 2012). From this initial, transverse segment emerges a branch for the caudate lobe. After the transverse course, the left portal vein turns 90 degrees anteriorly. This secondary segment of the left portal vein is located deep in the groove of the round ligament of the liver, and is termed the umbilical portion of the left portal vein. At the turning point of the left portal vein, between the transverse and umbilical segments inserts the ligamentum venosum of Arantii. The umbilical portion of the left portal vein may be covered by a bridge of liver parenchyma passing between segment 3 and 4, it can be, as thick as 2 cm, a thin fibrous band or even absent. In contrast to the right portal vein, neither portion of the left portal vein enters the hepatic substance, but rather lies directly on the surface (Strasberg, 2010). At the base of segment 4, the initial transverse segment of the left portal vein is accompanied by the left hepatic duct, the left hepatic artery joining the glissonian pedicle at the base of the umbilical fissure. From the left side of the umbilical segment of the left portal vein emerges the portal branch for segment 2 (usually only one), from its proximal part, and the portal branch for segment 3 (usually only one), from its distal part. From the right side emerges branches for segment 4 (usually more than one).

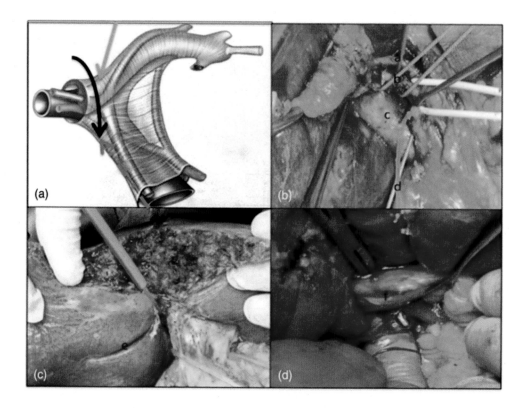

Figure 72. Selective pedicle clamping (extrahepatic, transhepatic and Glissonian). (a) Selective pedicle clamping. (b) Extrahepatic clamping. (c) Transhepatic clamping. (d) The Glissonian approach. a, hepatic artery; b, biliary duct; c, portal vein; d, transcystic drain; e, Rouviere's sulcus; f, right portal branch (Figure reproduced with permission from John Wiley and Sons from Charlotte Mouly, David Fuks, François Browet, François Mauvais, Arnaud Potier, Thierry Yzet, Qassemyar Quentin, Jean-Marc Regimbeau. Feasibility of the Glissonian approach during right hepatectomy. HPB – The Official Journal of the International Hepato Pancreato Biliary Association. 2013 15 (8), 638–645) (Mouly *et al.*, 2013).

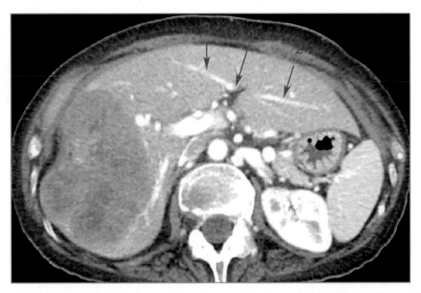

Figure 73. Computed Tomography, axial section, revealing the terminal portion of the umbilical segment of left portal vein (1) with segmental branches for segment 3 (2) and segment 4 (3) (Image courtesy of Radiology and Imagistics Department, Emergency Hospital of Bucharest).

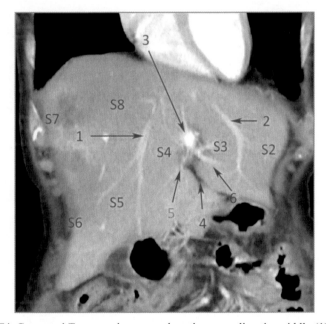

Figure 74. Computed Tomography, coronal section, revealing the middle (1) and left (2) hepatic veins. 3 – umbilical segment of the left portal vein (3), 4 – round ligament, 5 – P4, portal branch for segment 4, 6 – P3, portal branch for segment 3. S2, S3, S4, S5, S6, S7, S8 are liver segments (Image courtesy of Radiology and Imagistics Department, Emergency Hospital of Bucharest).

THE COMMON HEPATIC ARTERY

In the prevailing anatomy pattern the common hepatic artery has its origin in the celiac trunk, together with the splenic and left gastric arteries. After a short trajectory of 2–3 cm, inferiorly and to the right, above the upper margin of the first duodenum it divides into the proper hepatic and gastroduodenal arteries.

THE PROPER HEPATIC ARTERY

Around one third of the blood flow and half of the oxygen of the liver are brought by the proper hepatic artery. The proper hepatic artery, located anterior and to the left in the hepatoduodenal ligament, it divides after a course of 2–3 cm into a left and a right hepatic artery.

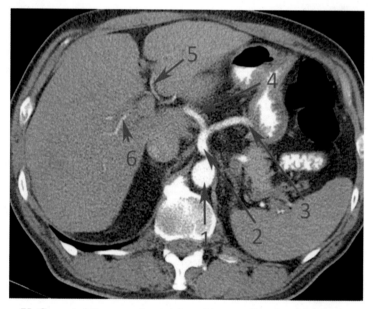

Figure 75. Computed Tomography, axial section, revealing the abdominal aorta (1), celiac artery (2), splenic artery (3), common hepatic artery (4), left (5) and right (6) hepatic arteries (Image courtesy of Radiology and Imagistics Department, Emergency Hospital of Bucharest).

The right hepatic artery, most commonly (80% of cases) has a trajectory posterior to the common hepatic duct. At this level, in Calot's hepatocystic triangle, emerges the cystic artery. The boundaries of Calot's triangle are the cystic duct, the common hepatic duct and the visceral surface of the liver. The right hepatic artery further divides into intraparenchymatous branches similar to the right portal vein.

The left hepatic artery has an ascending trajectory, entering into the liver parenchyma on the left side of the liver hilum. From is initial extra-parenchymal segment emerges an intermediate branch for segment 4. The caudate lobe usually receives two arteries, each branching off of the right and left hepatic arteries.

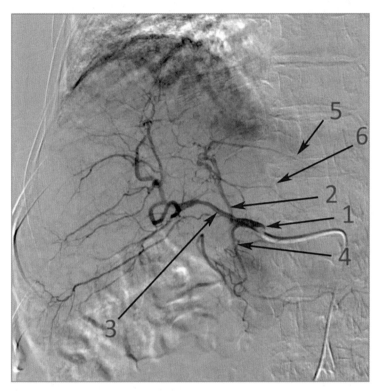

Figure 76. Angiography of the common hepatic artery (1) revealing the left hepatic artery (2) with segment 2 (5) and 3 (6) arterial branches, right hepatic artery (3), and gastroduodenal artery (4), (Figure courtesy of Emergency Hospital of Bucharest, Department of Angiography).

During hepatic surgery it is recommended not to make assumptions regarding the hepatic arteries based on size or position, but to rely instead on exposure, trial occlusion and preoperative imagistics (Strasberg, 2010). Approximately 25% of patients have a replaced or accessory hepatic artery. "Replaced" means that the artery has an unusual origin and represents the only arterial source for the respective area of the liver. "Accessory" means that the specific artery has an unusual origin, co-existing with a smaller artery with a normal origin and course. Hiatt et al. studied the anatomic variations in the hepatic arteries in 1000 patients who underwent liver harvesting for orthotopic liver transplantation (Hiatt, Gabbay and Busuttil, 1994).

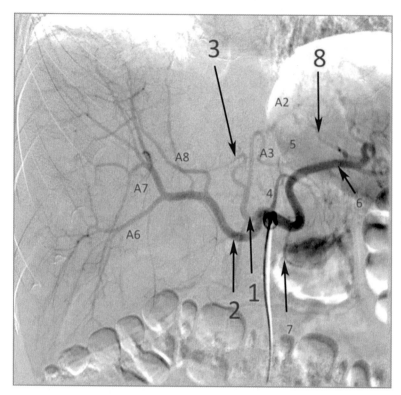

Figure 77. Angiography of the celiac artery revealing the left hepatic artery (1), right hepatic artery (2), splenic artery (6) with the dorsal pancreatic artery (7) and the posterior gastric artery (8), left gastric artery (4) with its cardiacoesophageal branch (5). 3 – A4, arterial branch from the left hepatic artery for segment 4, A2 – arterial branch from the left hepatic artery for segment 2, A3 – arterial branch from the left hepatic artery for segment 3, A6 – arterial branch from the right hepatic artery for segment 6, A7 – arterial branch from the right hepatic artery for segment 7, A8 – arterial branch from the right hepatic artery for segment 8 (Figure courtesy of Emergency Hospital of Bucharest, Department of Angiography).

Table 10
Pattern of hepatic arterial supply according to Hiatt *et al.* (Hiatt, Gabbay and Busuttil, 1994)

Arterial pattern	Frequency	Description
Type 1	75.7%	CHA arising from the CA, dividing into the GDA and PHA, PHA dividing into the LHA and RHA
Type 2	9.7%	Replaced or accessory LHA arising from the left gastric artery
Type 3	10.6%	Replaced or accessory right hepatic artery arising from SMA
Type 4	2.3%	RHA from SMA and LHA from left gastric artery
Type 5	1.5%	CHA from SMA
Type 6	0.2%	CHA from aorta

CHA – common hepatic artery; CA – celiac artery; GDA – gastroduodenal artery; PHA – proper hepatic artery; LHA – left hepatic artery; RHA – right hepatic artery; SMA – superior mesenteric artery.

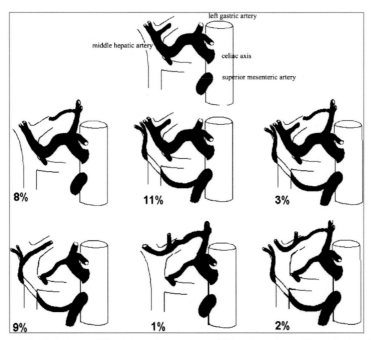

Figure 78. Variations of the 3 hepatic arteries: middle, from the celiac axis; left from the left gastric artery; right from the superior mesenteric artery [Figure reproduced with permission from John Wiley and Sons from Surgical anatomy of the biliary tract, Denis Castaign, HPB, 10 (2), 72–76, 2009 (Castaing, 2008)].

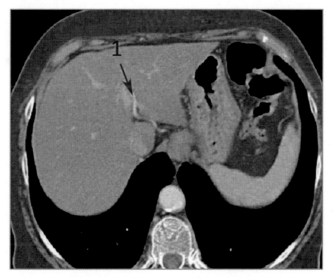

Figure 79. Computed Tomography, axial section, revealing a replaced left hepatic artery with the origin in the left gastric artery, travelling through the fissure of the venous ligament of Arantius, where it enters the the liver parenchyma (Image courtesy of Radiology and Imagistics Department, Emergency Hospital of Bucharest).

HEPATIC VEINS

There are three hepatic veins, right, middle and left, draining into the inferior vena cava. The right hepatic vein is located in the right intersectional plane, and has a short, around 1 cm, extrahepatic course.

The middle hepatic vein is located in the median intersectional plane. Analyzing the pattern of the middle hepatic vein distal branches in 20 patients with right hepatectomy with conservation of the middle hepatic vein, Faitot *et al.* found the classical pattern in 70%, 20% of patients had type B and 10% had type C pattern (Faitot *et al.*, 2012).

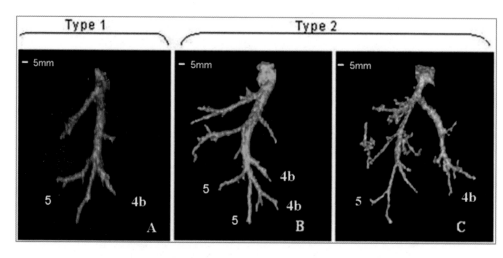

Figure 80. Middle hepatic vein (MHV) types according to the Renz–Neumann classification. (a) Type A consists of a classical disposition with bifurcation of the MHV trunk into two major tributaries for segments V and IVb. (b) Type B presents a long common trunk with multiple small tributaries draining segment IVb. (c) Type C has a short common trunk with a large IVb tributary passing through the parenchyma of segment IV [Figure reproduced with permission from Jon Wiley and Sons, from Francois Faitot, Eric Vibert, Chady Salloum, David Lee Gorden, Franck Coscas, René Adam, Denis Castaing. Importance of conserving middle hepatic vein distal branches for homogeneous right of the left liver after right hepatectomy. HPB – The Official Journal of the International Hepato Pancreato Biliary Association. 14 (11), 746–753, 2012 (Faitot *et al.*, 2012)].

The origin of the middle hepatic vein is immediately deep to the cystic plate. During cholecystectomy, if gallbladder dissection is performed deep to the cystic plate significant hemorrhage can occur.

The left hepatic vein begins between segments 2 and 3. It travels in this plane for most of its length. 1 cm from its convergence into the IVC, the left hepatic vein may be found in the left intersectional plane, where the "umbilical vein", which drains the left part of segment 4 is received (Strasberg, 2010; Hann, 2012). Usually the middle and left hepatic veins form at a distance of about 1 cm from the IVC, a common trunk.

In about 63–68% of cases may be found a right inferior hepatic vein, which drains segment 6 (Poston and Blumgart, 2003; Jones and Poston, 2011). There are a number of small hepatic veins, draining directly into the inferior vena cava from the caudate lobe.

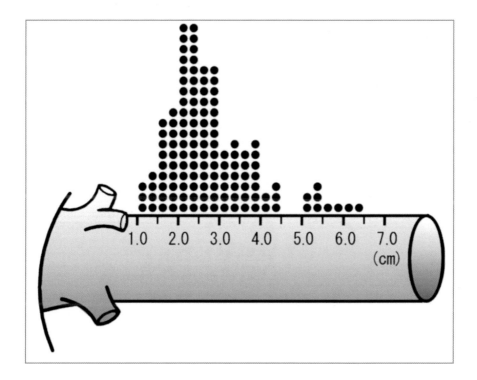

Figure 81. Schematic longitudinal view of the inferior vena cava showing the distribution of the caudate veins according to the distance between the caudal edge of the middle and left hepatic veins and the orifice of the typical caudate vein. Typical caudate veins were sorted into categories of 5-mm increments in this distance [Figure reproduced with permission from John Wiley and Sons with Nobuyuki Takemura, Kiyoshi Hasegawa, Yasuhiko Sugawara, Keming Zhang, Taku Aoki, Yoshifumi Beck, Masatoshi Makuuchi, Norihiro Kokudo. Morphometric analysis of caudate veins for advanced liver surgery. HPB – The Official Journal of the Inter-national Hepato Pancreato Biliary Association, 2010, 12 (9), 619–624, (Takemura *et al.*, 2010)].

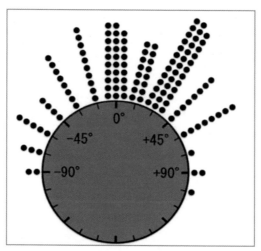

Figure 82. Distribution of 135 typical caudate veins detected by preoperative computed tomography with contrast material in transverse view. The surface of the inferior vena cava is schematically divided into intervals of 15° [Figure reproduced with permission from John Wiley and Sons with Nobuyuki Takemura, Kiyoshi Hasegawa, Yasuhiko Sugawara, Keming Zhang, Taku Aoki, Yoshifumi Beck, Masatoshi Makuuchi, Norihiro Kokudo. Morphometric analysis of caudate veins for advanced liver surgery. HPB – The Official Journal of the International Hepato Pancreato Biliary Association, 2010, 12 (9), 619–624, (Takemura *et al.*, 2010)].

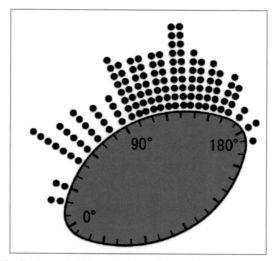

Figure 83. Distribution of 130 typical caudate veins detected by intraoperative ultrasound in transverse view. The surface of the inferior vena cava is schematically divided into intervals of 10° [Figure reproduced with permission from John Wiley and Sons with Nobuyuki Takemura, Kiyoshi Hasegawa, Yasuhiko Sugawara, Keming Zhang, Taku Aoki, Yoshifumi Beck, Masatoshi Makuuchi, Norihiro Kokudo. Morphometric analysis of caudate veins for advanced liver surgery. HPB – The Official Journal of the International Hepato Pancreato Biliary Association, 2010, 12 (9), 619–624, (Takemura *et al.*, 2010)].

RETROHEPATIC INFERIOR VENA CAVA

At the level of the renal veins, the inferior vena cava (IVC) is located posterior to the duodenum and pancreatic head, below Treitz's fascia. Above this level, it passes posterior to the foramen of Winslow, then having an ascending trajectory at the level of the bare area of the liver, in a manner determined by the hepatic parenchyma. The IVC traverses the diaphragm through the central tendon, at the level of the eighth thoracic vertebra. During its course, the retrohepatic IVC receives the right adrenal vein. Inferior to the right renal vein, the IVC receives on its posterolateral surface the lumbar veins, but above this level, usually there are no tributaries posteriorly (Hann, 2012).

LIVER SEGMENTATION

The functional surgical anatomy of the liver is determined by the intrahepatic distribution of biliary and vascular structures, which overlap only partially with the external configuration. Its understanding is the cornerstone of liver resections.

The intrahepatic distribution of the biliary and vascular elements, with consequent description of liver division, was masterfully presented by Ton That Tung, Healey and Schroy, Goldsmith and Woodburne, Couinaud and Bismuth (Tung, 1939, 1979; Healey, J.E., Schroy, 1953; Couinaud, 1957; Goldsmith, N.A., Woodburne, 1957; Bismuth, Houssin and Castaing, 1982). The most complete description was that proposed by Couinaud, which correlates with surgical liver resections. This classification divides the liver into anatomical units based on intrahepatic portal vein distribution (Couinaud, 1999).

The watersheds of the hepatic artery, the bile duct and the portal vein are identical, except for their second order division on the left side of the liver (Strasberg et al., 2000). The watersheds for arterial and biliary structures divide the left side of the liver via the umbilical fissure. The portal vein watershed divides the left side of the liver through a plane located between the segments 2 and 3. In an effort to internationally standardize the terminology of liver divisions, especially in published literature regarding liver resections, a committee of the International Hepato-Pancreatico-Biliary Association, chaired by Steven Strasberg, met in Brisbane, Australia in 2000, and proposed "The Brisbane 2000 Terminology of Liver Anatomy and Resections" (Strasberg et al., 2000). This terminology is based on intrahepatic distribution of arterial and biliary elements, and added the terminology of second-order division based on the portal vein, which is also anatomically correct as an addendum. The term for second-order division based on arterial and biliary watersheds is "section" (Healey and Schroy), while the term for second-order division based on portal vein distribution (Couinaud's concept) is "sector" (Strasberg et al., 2000).

	Volume, cm³, median (range)	% of total liver volume, median (range)
Total liver	1115 (775–2032)	
Left liver	354 (154–628)	31.2% (15.3–45.3%)
Right liver	701 (493–1324)	65.1% (50.3–75.5%)
Paramedian sector	415 (142–835)	38.5% (15.6–51.1%)
Lateral sector	290 (135–571)	26.3% (15.5–47.1%)
Segment I	45 (13–122)	4.0% (1.3–10.1%)
Segment II	90 (25–187)	7.9% (2.9–16.1%)
Segment III	106 (46–232)	9.5% (4.1–19.8%)
Segment IV	151 (51–262)	13.6% (5.1–20.9%)
Segment V	136 (41–249)	12.6% (4.4–20.0%)
Segment VI	87 (11–272)	7.9% (1.2–20.0%)
Segment VII	197 (69–501)	16.8% (6.0–35.8%)
Segment VIII	275 (101–586)	26.1% (11.1–38.0%)

Figure 84. Volumetric data obtained in 107 healthy livers [Table reproduced with permission from John Wiley and Sons, from Yoshihiro Mise, Shouichi Satou, Junichi Shindoh, Claudius Conrad, Taku Aoki, Kiyoshi Hasegawa, Yasuhiko Sugawara, Norihiro Kokudo. Three-dimensional volumetry in 107 normal livers reveals clinically relevant inter-segment variation in size. HPB – The Official Journal of the International Hepato Pancreato Biliary Associatio. 16 (5), 439–447, 2014 (Mise *et al.*, 2014)].

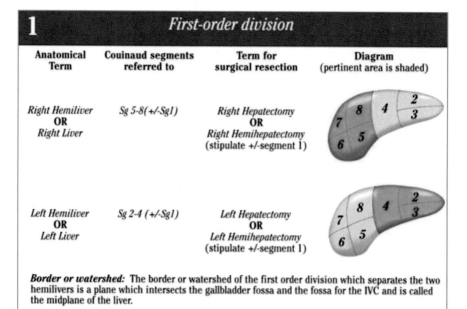

Figure 85. Schematic diagram of the two hemilivers (Figure reproduced with permission from John Wiley and Sons from The Brisbane 2000 Terminology of Liver Anatomy and Resections. Terminology Committee of the International Hepato-Pancreato-Biliary Association. HPB. 2000; 2 (3):333–39) (Strasberg *et al.*, 2000).

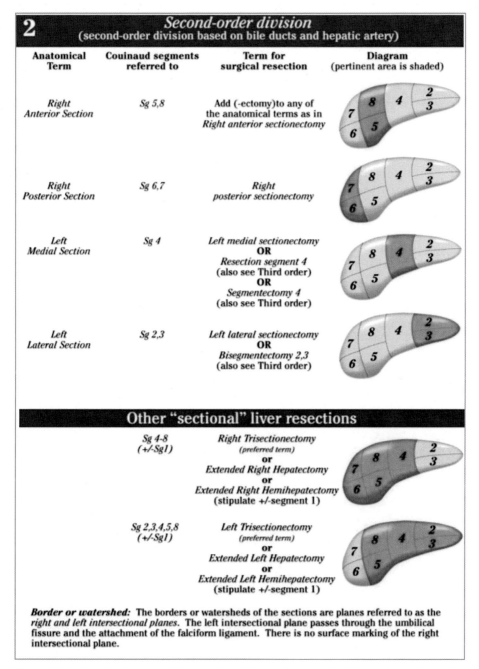

2 **Second-order division** (second-order division based on bile ducts and hepatic artery)			
Anatomical Term	**Couinaud segments referred to**	**Term for surgical resection**	**Diagram** (pertinent area is shaded)
Right Anterior Section	*Sg 5,8*	Add (-ectomy)to any of the anatomical terms as in *Right anterior sectionectomy*	
Right Posterior Section	*Sg 6,7*	*Right posterior sectionectomy*	
Left Medial Section	*Sg 4*	*Left medial sectionectomy* **OR** *Resection segment 4* (also see Third order) **OR** *Segmentectomy 4* (also see Third order)	
Left Lateral Section	*Sg 2,3*	*Left lateral sectionectomy* **OR** *Bisegmentectomy 2,3* (also see Third order)	
Other "sectional" liver resections			
	Sg 4-8 (+/-Sg1)	*Right Trisectionectomy* (*preferred term*) or *Extended Right Hepatectomy* or *Extended Right Hemihepatectomy* (stipulate +/-segment 1)	
	Sg 2,3,4,5,8 (+/-Sg1)	*Left Trisectionectomy* (*preferred term*) or *Extended Left Hepatectomy* or *Extended Left Hemihepatectomy* (stipulate +/-segment 1)	

Border or watershed: The borders or watersheds of the sections are planes referred to as the *right and left intersectional planes*. The left intersectional plane passes through the umbilical fissure and the attachment of the falciform ligament. There is no surface marking of the right intersectional plane.

Figure 86. Schematic diagram of the sections (Figure reproduced with permission from John Wiley and Sons from The Brisbane 2000 Terminology of Liver Anatomy and Resections. Terminology Committee of the International Hepato-Pancreato-Biliary Association. HPB. 2000; 2 (3):333–39) (Strasberg *et al.*, 2000).

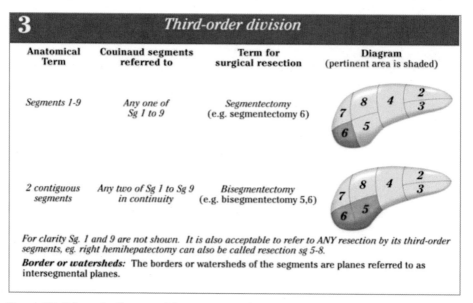

3	*Third-order division*		
Anatomical Term	**Couinaud segments referred to**	**Term for surgical resection**	**Diagram** (pertinent area is shaded)
Segments 1-9	*Any one of Sg 1 to 9*	*Segmentectomy* (e.g. segmentectomy 6)	
2 contiguous segments	*Any two of Sg 1 to Sg 9 in continuity*	*Bisegmentectomy* (e.g. bisegmentectomy 5,6)	

For clarity Sg. 1 and 9 are not shown. It is also acceptable to refer to ANY resection by its third-order segments, eg. right hemihepatectomy can also be called resection sg 5-8.

Border or watersheds: The borders or watersheds of the segments are planes referred to as intersegmental planes.

Figure 87. Schematic diagram of the segments (Figure reproduced with permission from John Wiley and Sons from The Brisbane 2000 Terminology of Liver Anatomy and Resections. Terminology Committee of the International Hepato-Pancreato-Biliary Association. HPB. 2000; 2 (3):333–39) (Strasberg *et al.*, 2000).

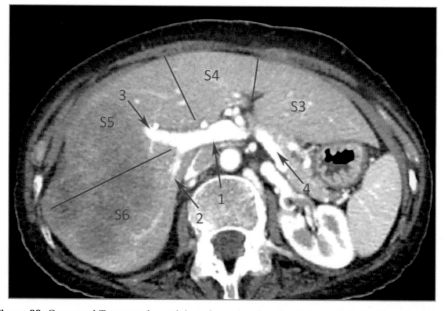

Figure 88. Computed Tomography, axial section, revealing the right portal vein (1) with its right posterior (2) and right anterior (3) sectional branches. 4 – splenic vein. S3, S4, S5 and S6 are liver segments (Image courtesy of Radiology and Imagistics Department, Emergency Hospital of Bucharest).

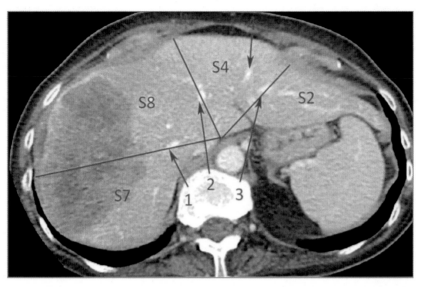

Figure 89. Computed Tomography, axial section, revealing the right (1), middle (2) and left (3) hepatic veins. 4 – umbilical vein, which drains into the left hepatic vein. If the left hepatic vein is located in the left portal fissure (between segment 2 and 3), the umbilical vein is located in the left intersectional plane (between segments 3 and 4). S2, S4, S8, S7 are liver segments. The anatomical limit between superior and inferior segments is represented by the right branch of the portal vein (Image courtesy of Radiology and Imagistics Department, Emergency Hospital of Bucharest).

It should be observed that segments are numbered with Arabic numerals, the Roman ones being unfamiliar to non-Western countries.

In conclusion, according to its functional anatomy, the liver may be divided into *right and left hemilivers*. The limit between these two anatomical units is represented by the *midplane of the liver*, which passes through the gallbladder fossa and IVC. The middle hepatic vein is located in the midplane of the liver.

The right hemiliver has *anterior and posterior sections*, which are separated by the *right intersectional plane*. The right intersectional plane has no external landmarks, and includes at its level the right hepatic vein. The anterior section includes segments 5 and 8. The posterior section includes segments 6 and 7.

The left hemiliver has *lateral and medial sections*, which are delimited by the *left intersectional plane*. The left intersectional plane passes through the umbilical fissure on the inferior liver surface and through the falciform ligament on the diaphragmatic surface of the liver. It should be noted that only the terminal segment of the left hepatic vein may be found in the left intersectional plane, its proximal part being located between segments 2 and 3. The medial section includes segment 4 and the lateral section includes segments 2 and 3.

4   **Addendum.** *Alternative second-order division*
(second-order division based on portal vein)

Anatomical Term	Couinaud segments referred to	Term for surgical resection	Diagram (pertinent area is shaded)
Right Anterior Sector OR *Right paramedian Sector*	*Sg 5,8*	Add (-ectomy)to any of the anatomical terms as in *Right anterior sectorectomy* OR *Right paramedian sectorectomy*	
Right Posterior Sector OR *Right Lateral Sector*	*Sg 6,7*	*Right posterior sectorectomy* OR *Right lateral sectorectomy*	
Left Medial Sector OR *Left Paramedian Sector*	*Sg 3,4*	*Left medial sectorectomy* OR *Left paramedian sectorectomy* OR *Bisegmentectomy 3,4*	
Left Lateral Sector OR *Left Posterior Sector*	*Sg 2*	*Left lateral sectorectomy* OR *Left posterior sectorectomy* OR *Segmentectomy 2*	

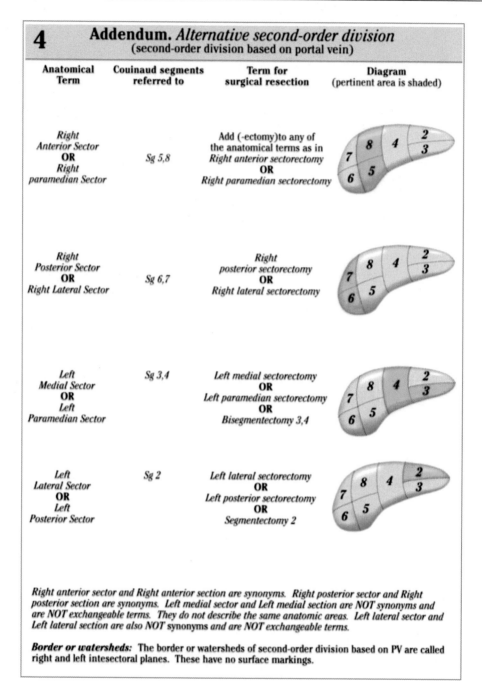

Right anterior sector and Right anterior section are synonyms. Right posterior sector and Right posterior section are synonyms. Left medial sector and Left medial section are NOT synonyms and are NOT exchangeable terms. They do not describe the same anatomic areas. Left lateral sector and Left lateral section are also NOT synonyms and are NOT exchangeable terms.

Border or watersheds: The border or watersheds of second-order division based on PV are called right and left intesectoral planes. These have no surface markings.

Figure 90. Schematic diagram of the second-order division based on the portal vein (Figure reproduced with permission from John Wiley and Sons from The Brisbane 2000 Terminology of Liver Anatomy and Resections. Terminology Committee of the International Hepato-Pancreato-Biliary Association. HPB. 2000; 2 (3):333–39) (Strasberg *et al.*, 2000).

In 2013, Strasberg and Phillips evaluated the use and dissemination of the Brisbane 2000 nomenclature 10 years after its introduction (Strasberg and Phillips, 2013). The use of the terms "right and left hemihepatectomy/hepatectomy" increased dramatically after the terminology was introduced, to the detriment of "right and left lobectomy". In the Americas and Asia the usage of these terms increased from less than 50% in papers published between 1990–1999 to 80% in papers as of 2006. The authors concluded that the Brisbane terminology is being adopted worldwide but its adoption is still incomplete (Strasberg and Phillips, 2013).

THE CAUDATE LOBE

The caudate lobe, or segment 1, represents the dorsal portion of the liver, located posterior to the left portal triad and anterior to the retrohepatic IVC.

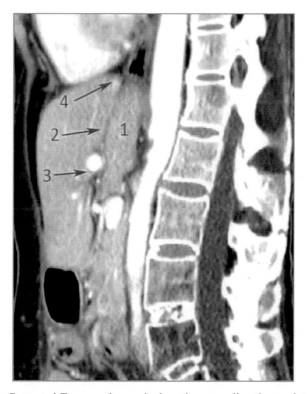

Figure 91. Computed Tomography, sagittal section, revealing the caudate lobe (1). 2 – the fissure of the venous ligament of Arantius, which connects left portal vein (3) with the left hepatic vein (4) (Image courtesy of Radiology and Imagistics Department, Emergency Hospital of Bucharest).

The caudate lobe is anatomically and functionally separate from the rest of the liver, since its vascularization is independent of the portal vein divisions and of the three main hepatic veins (Poston and Blumgart, 2003).

The anterior surface of the caudate lobe continues with the posterior surface of segment 4, the limit between these two structures being an oblique plane which passes through the left portal vein inferiorly and through the left hepatic vein, superiorly.

The caudate lobe may be divided according to Kumon into three parts (Peng, 2010):

The Spigelian lobe, the main bulk of the caudate lobe, located to the left of the IVC, being separated from the inferior surface of segments 2 and 3 by the lesser omentum. This part of the caudate lobe is free in the omental bursa.

The paracaval portion, located just in front of the IVC.

The caudate process, an elongation of the caudate lobe which extends to the inferior surface of segment 6, located between the left portal vein (anteriorly) and the IVC groove (posteriorly).

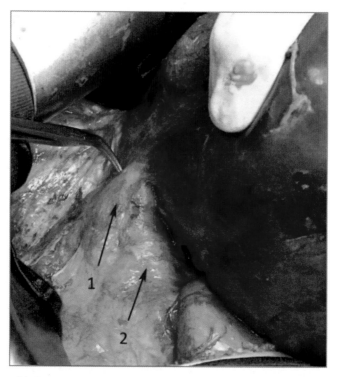

Figure 92. Intraoperative view of the hepatocaval ligament (1) and retrohepatic inferior vena cava (2) (Image from personal collection of IN).

According to Couinaud, the caudate lobe is subdivided into two parts, with the middle hepatic vein as a landmark (Abdalla, Vauthey and Couinaud, 2002):

Left part, segment I

Right part, segment IX

The left segment of the caudate lobe is continued by a fibrous component, which surrounds the IVC, ending on the posterior surface of segment 7. This hepatocaval ligament, also called Makuuchi's ligament, is not simple connective tissue, but rather contains vascular and biliary elements, which require surgical control (suture or stapling) during liver mobilization.

The vascular supply of the caudate lobe is through direct branches from the right and left portal triad, while biliary drainage is directly into the right and left bile ducts. The small arteries originate directly from the right and left hepatic artery. The portal vein branches are variable: 2–6 vessels come from the left portal vein, 2–3 come from the right portal vein and 1–2 come from the portal vein bifurcation (Guglielmi, Ruzzenente and Iacono, 2008).

The venous drainage of the caudate lobe is made directly into the IVC, and not through the hepatic veins. Takemura *et al*. analyzed the anatomic distribution of caudate veins in 116 donor hepatectomies for adult living donor liver transplantation (Takemura et al., 2010). In 116 patients were detected 152 caudate veins, which were typical in 135 cases and non-typical in 17 cases. One caudate vein was detected in 72%, two in 26% and three in 3%. 67% of caudate veins detected by intraoperative ultrasonography and 70% of those detected by CT were located on the ventral 60 degrees of the inferior vena cava. The remaining veins were scattered on both lateral sides (Takemura *et al*., 2010). In Budd-Chiari syndrome, when all three main hepatic veins are occluded, the liver venous return is accomplished through the caudate veins. In this scenario, the caudate lobe undergoes compensatory hypertrophy.

PLATE AND SHEATH SYSTEM OF THE LIVER

The plate and sheath of the liver is represented by fibrous tissue, which forms on the inferior surface of the liver's four plates:

Hilar

Cystic

Umbilical

Arantian

These plates are continued into the liver parenchyma with tubular structures which cover the glissonian (or portal) pedicles, termed sheaths. The hilar plate is represented by connective tissue located posterior and superior from the vascular and biliary structures located in the liver hilum (even from the right and left hepatic ducts, which are the most cranial structures in the liver hilum). The right portal pedicle is surrounded by a fibrous sheath once it enters into the liver parenchyma. The left portal pedicle is not surrounded by a fibrous sheath, only the segmental branches are surrounded by a fibrous sheath (Strasberg, 2010).

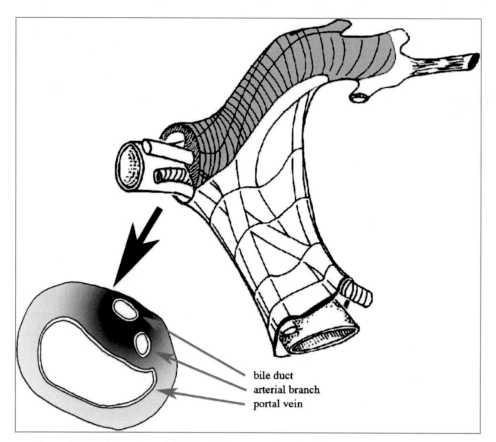

bile duct
arterial branch
portal vein

Figure 93. The hilar plate of the liver (Figure reproduced with permission from John Wiley and Sons from Surgical anatomy of the biliary tract, Denis Castaign, HPB, 10 (2), 72–76, 2009 (Castaing, 2008)).

The cystic plate is represented by the connective tissue located between the upper surface of the gallbladder and the liver parenchyma. The umbilical plate is located above the umbilical segment of the left portal vein.

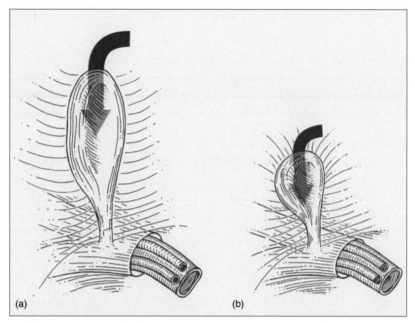

Figure 94. The relationship between the cystic plate and the right portal pedicle (a) under normal circumstances and (b) in the presence of severe contractive inflammation. The cystic plate attaches to the anterior surface of the right portal pedicle. Dissection downward in the plane deep to the plate (arrow) will lead to the pedicle, with injury to the vessels and bile duct. When inflammation is mild, as in (a), entry into the plane is usually readily detected by visualization of liver tissue. When there is severe contractive inflammation the cystic plate is thickened, as in (b), and determining the position of the dissection in relation to the plate is difficult. In addition, the plate is foreshortened so that the distance from the top of the plate to the pedicle is very short. Both of these factors greatly increase the likelihood of injury to the pedicle [Figure reproduced with permission from John Willey and Sons from Steven Strasberg, Dirk Gouma. "Extreme" vasculobiliary injuries: association with fundus-down cholecystectomy in severely inflamed gallbladders. HPB. 14 (1), 1–8, 2012 (Strasberg and Gouma, 2012)].

THE LYMPHATIC DRAINAGE

The origin of the hepatic lymphatic capillaries is in the perisinusoidal space of Disse. From this level, the lymphatic drainage is accomplished through a superficial and a deep pathway. The superficial lymphatics are located immediately beneath the Glisson's capsule. From here the lymph drains into the inferior vena cava lymph nodes, thoracic duct, hepatoduodenal lymph nodes, and pericardial lymph nodes. The deep lymphatic pathway traverses the liver parenchyma, draining superiorly into the IVC lymph nodes and inferiorly into the hepatoduodenal lymph nodes.

THE INNERVATION

The liver has sympathetic and parasympathetic innervation through the hepatic plexus. The hepatic plexus receives nervous fibers from the celiac plexus, with their trajectory around the hepatic artery and portal vein. In the hepatic plexus are coming parasympathetic fibers from the anterior and posterior vagal trunks. The liver Glisson's capsule receives somatic innervation, from the lower intercostal nerves. The diaphragmatic surface of the liver receives fibers from the right phrenic nerve, explaining the radiation of pain from biliary colic towards the right shoulder.

CHAPTER 17

HISTOLOGY

SORIN HOSTIUC, DANIELA STAN, REGINA KIRBY

Histologically the liver must be analyzed as being comprised of three main structures: the hepatic vascular system, the biliary tree and the 3D arrangement of the liver cells. Most blood enters into the liver through the portal system (around 75%), only 25% being arterial blood. The biliary system contains a series of channels and ducts whose main purpose is to lead the secreted bile to the lumen of the small intestine. The 3D architecture of the liver cells is maintained by a connective tissue matrix that starts at the Glisson capsule and branches into the inside of the organ. The structural unit of the liver is called the hepatic lobule, and it contains hexagonal rows of hepatocytes radiating from a central vein.

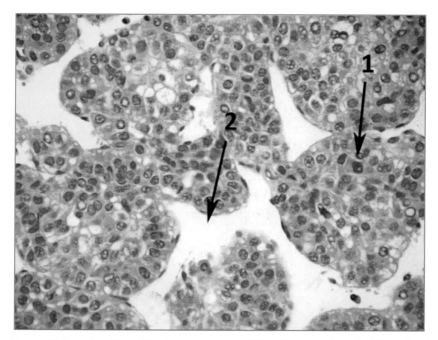

Figure 95. Hematoxylin and Eosin staining using 200 × objective of a well-differentiated hepatocellular carcinoma (1). 2 – sinusoid capillaries
(Image courtesy of VE, used with permission).

Liver steatosis (Fatty liver) is considered a reversible form of liver damage, associated with the accumulation of lipids in hepatocytes. The most common causes are alcohol abuse (that is associated with decreased NAD concentration in hepatocytes, the co-enzyme needed for hepatic lipolysis), and obesity. If the predisposing factors act continuously, it can lead to chronic hepatitis.

Chronic hepatitis is characterized by chronic inflammation of the liver. It is usually caused by viral agents (Hepatitis B or C), chronic alcohol abuse (alcoholic hepatitis), or by autoimmune processes. Histologically there are many forms of chronic hepatitis, the most common being:

• Chronic hepatitis with piecemeal necrosis (interface hepatitis), with or without fibrosis

• Chronic hepatitis without piecemeal necrosis (chronic persistent hepatitis).

Liver cirrhosis is characterized by the replacement of normal liver tissue with fibrous tissue and regenerating nodules. Initially the liver is enlarged but in later stages it decreases in size. Depending on the size of the nodules there are three main types of cirrhosis: micronodular (Laennec, portal), with nodules under 3 mm in diameter, mixed, and macronodular, the latter having mainly nodules larger than 3 mm.

Cholestasis is characterized by a decrease/arrest in the bile secretion and bile flow, being determined by either a functional secretory disturbance or by an obstruction in the billiary channels. It can be classified (Schaffner and Popper, 1985; Cullen, 2005):

• Depending on the location:
    – Intrahepatic – pathologies causing cholestasis located mainly inside the liver
    – Extrahepatic – pathologies causing cholestasis located mainly outside the liver.
• Depending on the severity:
    – Complete – usually associated with a complete arrest of bile secretion
    – Incomplete – usually caused by mechanical obstruction of the billiary channels or due to destructive diseases.
• Depending on the evolution:
    – Acute
    – Chronic

Primary biliary cirrhosis is an autoimmune disease characterized by the presence of chronic, destructive cholangitis ending in cirrhosis (Selmi et al., 2011).

Primary sclerosing cholangitis is characterized by the presence of pleomorphic and fibrous-obliterative cholangitis, having as a pathognomonic sign, onion-skin type periductal fibrosis, with degeneration and atrophy of the epithelium (Hirschfield et al., 2013).

Large ductal obstruction is caused by gallstones, tumors of ductal structures, tumors from the surrounding tissues (pancreas), etc. It is characterized by signs of acute complete cholestasis and can lead to secondary biliary cirrhosis.

Wilson disease (hepatolenticular degeneration) is caused by copper overload, and leads to hepatic cirrhosis early in life.

Hemosiderosis is caused by chronic anemia, chronic blood transfusions, hemolysis, chronic renal failure, genetic hemochromatosis, etc. It is easy to objectify using Pearls stain, which identifies Iron deposits, by the presence of an intense blue color (Nair, Fischer and Adeyi, 2010).

SECTION VII – THE EXTRAHEPATIC BILE DUCTS

Life is what happens while you are busy making other plans.

John Lennon

CHAPTER 18
EMBRYOLOGY

RUXANDRA IRINA NEGOI, SORIN PĂUN

The embryological development of the biliary tract is completed in close correlation with the liver, originating from the liver bud.

It is important to be familiar with anomalies of the extrahepatic bile ducts, to decrease the rate of iatrogenic injuries in this area.

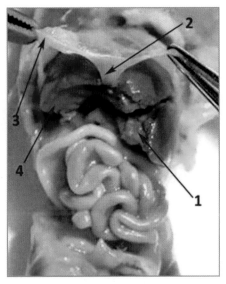

Figure 96. Anatomical dissection of a human embryo demonstrating the left-sided gallbladder (1), the falciform ligament (2), the diaphragm (3), and the liver (4) (Figure courtesy of RIN).

One important congenital malformation is gallbladder agenesis. The "ducts of Luschka" are small accessory bile ducts which drain the gallbladder directly into the liver, traversing the cystic plate. Their transection during cholecystectomy may produce postoperative biliary leakage.

Another very important anatomical variation with major impact on biliary surgery is low insertion of the right sectional hepatic ducts. In around 2% of patients, the right sectional duct, usually posterior sectional duct, joins the common hepatic duct just superior to the usual position of the cystic duct.

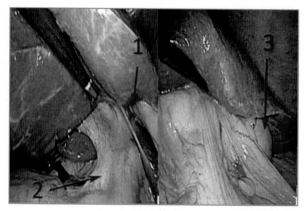

Figure 97. Intraoperative view of a left sided gallbladder: 1 – umbilical fissure of the liver, 2 – common bile duct (CBD), 3 – gallbladder on the left side of the CBD and round ligament of the liver (Image courtesy of IL and ML, used with permission).

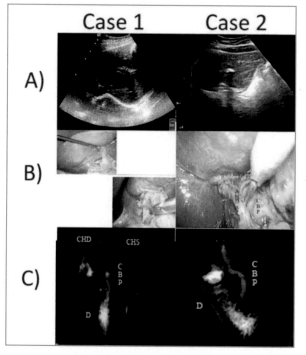

Figure 98. Two cases of gallbladder agenesis managed in the Emergency Hospital of Bucharest. A) preoperative ultrasonography, B) Intraoperative view with surgical dissection of the hepatoduodenal ligament. In Case 2 can be observed a replaced right hepatic artery (AHDA) with the origin in the superior mesenteric artery. C) One month postoperative MRCP. CHD, CHS – right and left hepatic ducts, CBP – common bile duct, D – duodenum (Image reproduced with permission from M. Beuran, S. Păun, I. Negoi, R. Gănescu, A. Runcanu, M. Avram, Al.L. Chiotoroiu. Abordul laparoscopic în agenezia veziculei biliare – o surpriză intraoperatorie. Chirurgia, 105 (4), 2010, 531–536).

CHAPTER 19
ANATOMY

IONUȚ NEGOI, MIRCEA BEURAN

The biliary ducts are divided, for didactic purposes, into an intrahepatic and an extrahepatic bile system. The extrahepatic bile ducts include the common bile duct and the accessory system (gallbladder and the cystic duct). Successful biliary surgery is based on (a) resection of all pathological tissue; (b) maintenance of adequate blood supply for the transected biliary margin; (c) maximal and effective drainage of the biliary tree (Poston and Blumgart, 2003).

INTRAHEPATIC BILE DUCTS

The intrahepatic biliary system has its origin at the level of the hepatic lobule. Initially, the intralobular hepatic ducts do not present walls, instead being bounded by the surfaces of the hepatocytes.

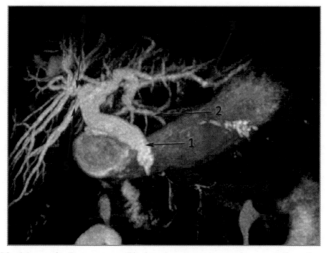

Figure 99. Magnetic Resonance Cholangiopancreatography revealing the common bile duct (1). 2 – segmentary bile duct from S3, segmentary bile duct from S2 (3). 4 – anterior sectional bile duct (from S5 ad S8), 5 – posterior sectional bile duct (from S6 and S8) (Image courtesy of Radiology and Imagistics Department, Emergency Hospital of Bucharest).

To the periphery of the hepatic lobule they gain walls, being called Hering's channels. They will converge as interlobular, segmental and sectional, up to the right and left hepatic ducts in the liver hilum. Prior to merging and giving rise to the right hepatic duct, the right anterior sectional duct has a vertical descending trajectory, while the right posterior sectional duct has a horizontal course.

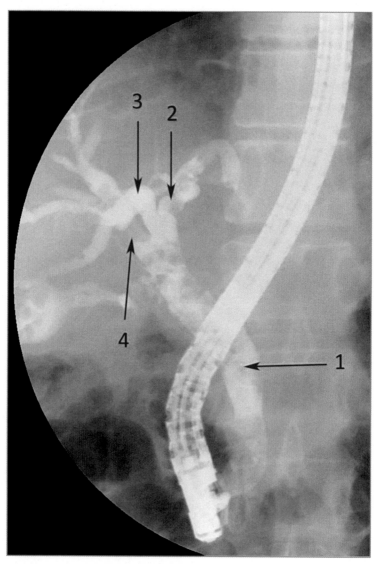

Figure 100. Endoscopic Retrograde Cholangiopancreatography revealing the common bile duct (1), the right posterior (3) sectional duct joining the left hepatic duct (2) and the right anterior sectional duct (4) (Image courtesy of GC, Gastroenterology Department, Emergency Hospital of Bucharest).

COMMON HEPATIC DUCT

The right and left hepatic ducts join together in the right extremity of the liver hilum, superior and anterior to the portal vein bifurcation, giving rise to the common hepatic duct. The common hepatic duct has a mean diameter of 4 mm, with a variable length of between one to seven centimeters. Usually, the common hepatic duct is located lateral to the left hepatic artery and anterior to the portal vein. Most frequently, related to the common hepatic duct, the right hepatic artery has a posterior trajectory.

Table 11
Biliary duct variation from classical distribution
(Healey, J.E., Schroy, 1953; Couinaud, 1957)

Hepatic ducts distribution	Couinaud	Healy and Schroy
Prevailing pattern	57%	72%
Triple confluence of the right posterior, right anterior and LHD	12%	–
Right sectional duct joining the CBD	Right anterior – 16% Right posterior – 4%	
Right sectional duct joining the LHD	Right anterior – 1% Right posterior – 5%	
Absence of the ducts confluence – all the sectional ducts joining separately	3%	
Right posterior duct joining the cystic duct or the gallbladder neck	2%	
Ectopic drainage of segment 5		9%
Ectopic drainage of segment 6		14%
Ectopic drainage of segment 8		20%
Subvesical duct (embedded in the cystic plate)		20–50%

CBD – common bile duct, LHD – left hepatic duct, RHA – right hepatic duct.

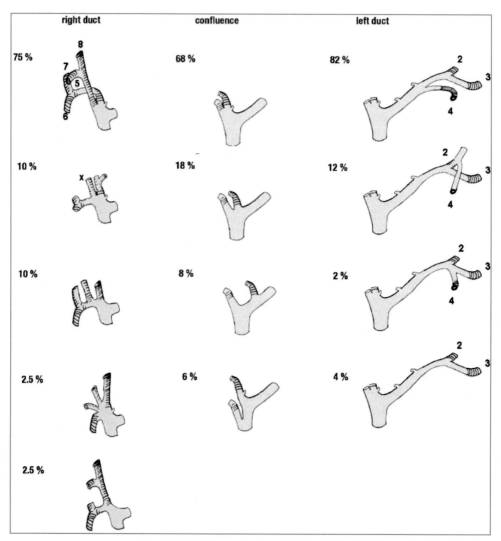

Figure 101. Intrahepatic duct and biliary confluence anatomy [Figure reproduced with permission from John Wiley and Sons from Surgical anatomy of the biliary tract, Denis Castaign, HPB, 10 (2), 72–76, 2009 (Castaing, 2008)].

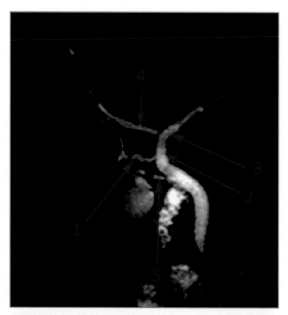

Figure 102. Magnetic Resonance Cholangiopancreatography, revealing low insertion of the right posterior sectional duct (1) into the common hepatic duct (2). 3 – left hepatic duct, 4 – right anterior sectional duct, 5 – cystic duct (Image courtesy of Radiology and Imagistics Department, Emergency Hospital of Bucharest).

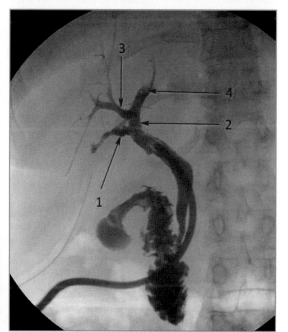

Figure 103. Endoscopic Retrograde Cholangiopancreatography revealing low insertion of the right posterior sectional duct (1) into the common hepatic duct (2). 3 – right anterior sectional duct, 4 – left hepatic duct (Image from Collection of Gastroenterology Department, Emergency Hospital of Bucharest).

GALLBLADDER

The gallbladder has a length of about 7–10 cm and a capacity of about 30–50 ml (Negoi *et al.*, 2010). It is located on the visceral surface of the liver, in the gallbladder fossa, between segments 4 and 5. The gallbladder is separated from the liver parenchyma through Glisson's capsule, termed at this level the cystic plate. The peritoneum from its inferior surface continues with the peritoneum from the visceral surface of the liver. The gallbladder may be divided topographically into the fundus, the body and the neck. The fundus is located 1–2 cm lower than the inferior edge of the liver, in close contact with the anterior abdominal wall. During clinical examination, the gallbladder fundus can be palpated in the cystic point. This is located at the intersection of the right costal margin with the lateral border of the right rectus abdominis muscle. The gallbladder's body has its upper surface in contact with the gallbladder fossa of the liver. Its inferior surface, covered by peritoneum, has anatomical relationships with the descending duodenum and transverse colon. At the level of the cystic plate, can be found the accessory portal veins of Sappey, a gallbladder vein being rarely present.

The gallbladder neck is located medially, in close anatomical relationships with the hepatic hilum and the right border of the hepatoduodenal ligament. The cystic artery is located in the connective tissue between the liver and the bladder neck. The mucosa of the neck presents transverse folds which form a spiral groove. This spiral groove is continued with the spiral valve of the cystic duct (Heister's valve). The gallbladder neck presents an inferior dilation, termed Hartmann's pouch. The hepatocystic triangle, delimited by the common hepatic duct (medially), the cystic duct (inferiorly) and the inferior surface of the liver (superiorly) is an important anatomical space, especially during laparoscopic cholecystectomy. In this area are usually found the cystic artery and Mascagni's lymph node. The hepatocystic triangle has several eponyms, such as Calot's triangle, which are confusing and should be abandoned (Strasberg, 2010). Steven Strasberg described "the critical view of safety" during laparoscopic cholecystectomy, which assumes clearance of the hepatocystic triangle, isolation of the cystic duct, and dissection with lowering of the gallbladder infundibulum from the cystic plate *(Vettoretto et al.*; Strasberg, Hertl and Soper, 1995). The "critical view of safety" is obtained if the operating surgeon can observe the inferior surface of the right hemiliver through the dissected hepatocystic triangle. In about 10% of cases, deep to the cystic plate may be found a large bile duct, its injury may cause significant biliary leakage.

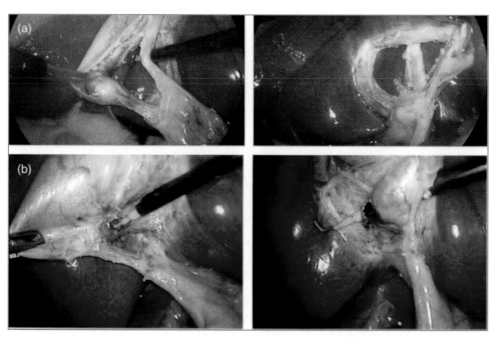

Figure 104. (a) Example of an "adequate" critical view of safety photo. (b) Example of an "inadequate" critical view of safety photo [Image reproduced with permission from John Wiley and Sons, from Tracey Lam, Val Usatoff, Steven T.F. Chan. Are we getting the critical view? A prospective study of photographic documentation during laparoscopic cholecystectomy. HPB, 16 (9), 859–863, 2014 (Lam, Usatoff and Chan, 2014)].

CYSTIC DUCT

The cystic duct connects the gallbladder with the common hepatic duct. It is about 3–4 cm long and 2–3 mm in width, it joins the common hepatic duct to form the common bile duct. Although the presence of two cystic ducts has been described, these anomalies are extremely rare. When a surgeon faces "two cystic ducts" during hepatocystic triangle dissection, these are usually the common bile duct and the common hepatic duct which were transected.

The mucosa of the cystic duct presents transverse folds, which give rise to the spiral valve of Heister. These spiral folds prevent the introduction of exploratory tools during surgical evaluation of the common bile duct.

The are three types of unions between the cystic and the common hepatic duct:

Angular type (60–70%): the cystic duct joins the common hepatic duct in an acute angle.

Parallel type (20%): the cystic duct has a longer parallel trajectory with the common hepatic duct, joining it distally.

Helicoidally (10%): the cystic duct passes anterior or posterior to the common hepatic duct, joining it on its left side.

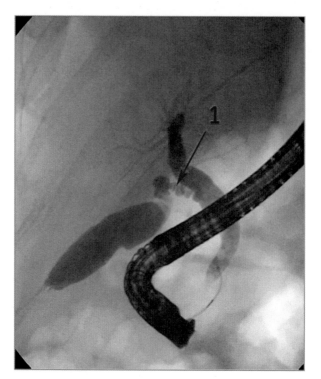

Figure 105. Endoscopic Retrograde Cholangiopancreatography revealing the filling defects produced by the Heister spiral valves (1) at the level of the cystic duct (Image from Collection of GC, Gastroenterology Department, Emergency Hospital of Bucharest).

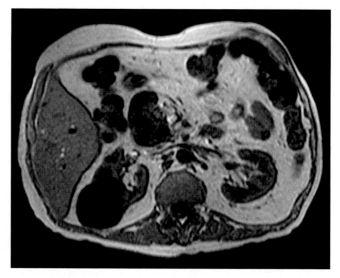

Figure 106. Magnetic Resonance Imaging revealing an Ampulla of Vater malignancy (Image courtesy of Emergency Hospital of Bucharest, used with permission).

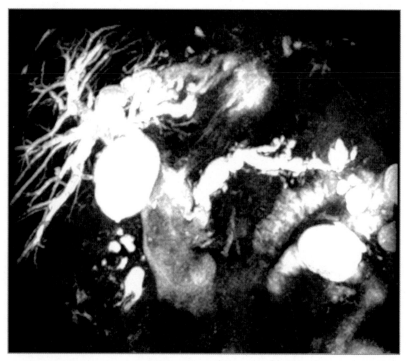

Figure 107. Magnetic Resonance Cholangiopancreatography (MRCP) revealing an Ampulla of Vater malignancy (Image courtesy of Emergency Hospital of Bucharest, used with permission).

COMMON BILE DUCT

The common bile duct has a length of 5–15 cm, with a mean diameter of 6 mm. During surgery, in patients with a long period of fasting, the common hepatic duct can be as narrow as 3 mm, which makes its reconstruction extremely difficult in the case of iatrogenic injury. A diameter greater than 8 mm suggests dilation of the common bile duct. Topographically it can be divided into four segments: supraduodenal, retroduodenal, retropancreatic and intramural. The supra-duodenal segment is located in the hepatoduodenal ligament, anterior to the portal vein and to the right of the proper hepatic artery. The retroduodenal segment is located posterior to the first part of the duodenum. Here, it has anatomical relationships with the portal vein (posteriorly) and the gastroduodenal artery (on its left). The superior posterior pancreaticoduodenal artery passes anteriorly to this segment. The retropancreatic segment is located posterior to the pancreatic head, in a groove or channel in its parenchyma. On its left it has relationships with the portal vein.

Posterior to Treitz's fascia the retropancreatic common bile duct has anatomical relationships with the left renal vein and the inferior vena cava. The superior posterior pancreaticoduodenal artery may be found in close posterior relationship with this common bile duct segment. It has a posterior trajectory. The last segment of the common bile duct is the intramural one, about 1.5 cm long, located in the medial wall of the descending duodenum. Its trajectory gives rise to a folding of the duodenal mucosa. At this level the bile duct joins the main pancreatic duct of Wirsung. There are three anatomical variants for the joining of the common bile duct to the main pancreatic duct:

They join together forming the hepatopancreatic ampulla of Vater.

They join just before the duodenum, without giving rise to the ampulla.

They have a parallel trajectory, opening separately into the duodenum.

Most commonly they form the hepatopancreatic ampulla of Vater. It opens on the posterior and medial wall of the descending duodenum, between the upper two thirds and the lower one third.

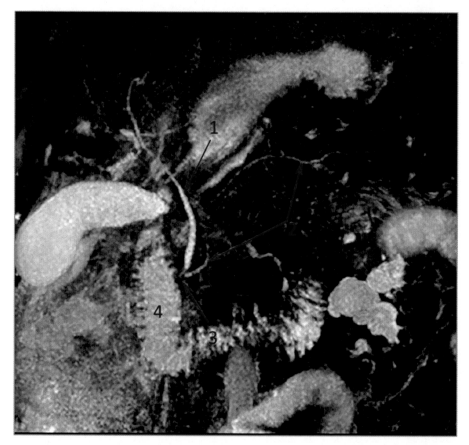

Figure 108. Magnetic Resonance Cholangiopancreatography, revealing the common bile duct (1) joining the main pancreatic duct (2) to form the ampulla of Vater (3). 4 – descending duodenum (Image courtesy of Radiology and Imagistics Department, Emergency Hospital of Bucharest).

The muscular sphincter of the hepatopancreatic ampulla was described for the first time by Oddi. He described a unitary sphincter, derived from the duodenal muscular wall. Subsequently, Boyden described a biliary duct sphincter and an ampulla sphincter, derived from the local mesenchyme. The sphincter was divided into three areas by Baraya. The junction between the middle and the lower segments is the narrowest zone.

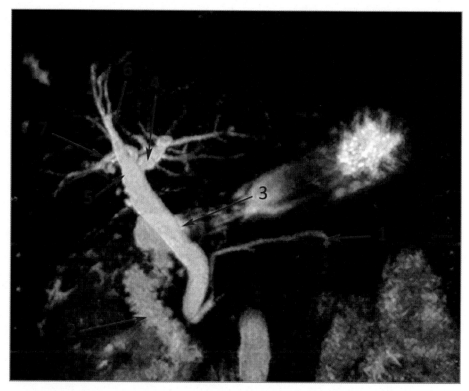

Figure 109. Magnetic Resonance Cholangiopancreatography revealing the pancreatic duct (1). 2 – duodenum, 3 – common bile duct, 4 – left hepatic duct, 5 – right hepatic duct, 6 – right anterior sectional biliary duct, 7 – right posterior sectional biliary duct (Image courtesy of Radiology and Imagistics Department, Emergency Hospital of Bucharest).

VASCULAR SUPPLY

ARTERIES

The arterial vascularization of the extrahepatic biliary ducts is represented by the neighboring arteries.

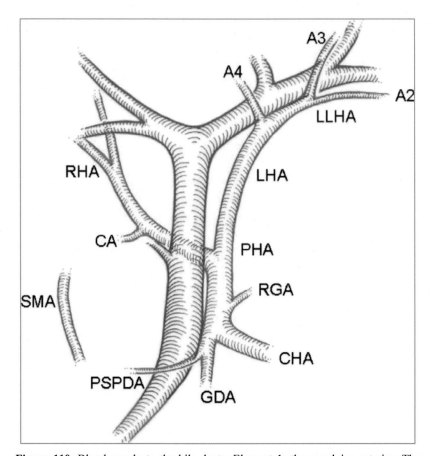

Figure 110. Blood supply to the bile ducts. Element 1: the supplying arteries. The arteries shown can all branch to the marginal arteries or, in some cases, directly supply the epicholedochal plexus. SMA, superior mesenteric artery; PSPDA, posterior superior pancreatoduodenal artery (the most important and constant artery); CHA, common hepatic artery; PHA, proper hepatic artery; RGA, right gastric artery; GDA, gastroduodenal artery; RHA, right hepatic artery; LHA, left hepatic artery; CA, cystic artery; LLHA, left lateral hepatic artery; A2, A3, A4, arteries to segments 2, 3 and 4. Replaced arteries can also supply the bile ducts [Figure reproduced with permission from John Wiley and Sons from Steven M. Strasberg,W. Scott Helton. An analytical review of vasculobiliary injury in laparoscopic and open cholecystectomy. HPB – The Official Journal of the International Hepato Pancreato Biliary Association. 13 (1), 1–14, 2011 (Strasberg and Helton, 2011)].

The cystic artery branches off, usually from the right hepatic artery, and can be found in the hepatocystic triangle. A useful anatomical landmark to identify the cystic artery during laparoscopic cholecystectomy is the Mascagni's lymph node, which is located just anteriorly. Medial to the gallbladder neck, the cystic artery branches off into an anterior and a posterior branch. In 15% of cases there are variations in the cystic artery origin, such as, the right hepatic artery crossing the anterior surface of the common hepatic duct, the replaced right hepatic artery coming off the superior mesenteric artery, the proper hepatic artery, or the gastroduodenal artery.

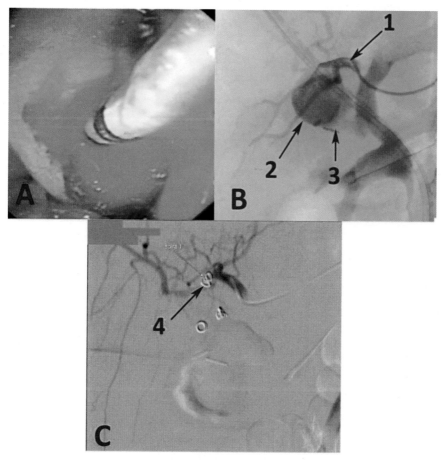

Figure 111. Hemobilia in a 46 year old female patient, seven months after a laparoscopic cholecystectomy: A – upper endoscopy image of blood exteriorization from the ampulla of Vater. B – angiography of the right hepatic artery (1) revealing a pseudo aneurism (2) and the metallic clips after cholecystectomy, C – angiographic aspect after selective embolization with metallic coils (4) (Image courtesy of MB, AC, used with permission).

A very dangerous anatomical conformation of the right hepatic artery in the hepatocystic triangle is its looping in this area, with the cystic artery emerging from the tip of the loop. This anatomical conformation predisposes to confusion of the right hepatic with the cystic artery, when clipping and transection.

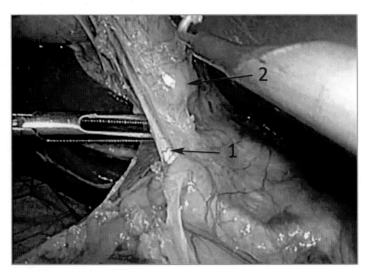

Figure 112. Intraoperative view of a cystic artery (1) originating into the gastroduodenal artery. 2 – gallbladder neck (Image courtesy of LM and SP, used with permission).

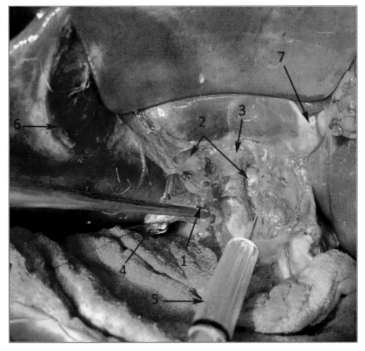

Figure 113. Intraoperative view of a cystic artery (1) with its origin in the right hepatic artery (2), which crosses the posterior surface of the common hepatic duct (3), then loops into the hepatocystic triangle. 4 – transected cystic duct, 5 – tourniquet used for Pringle maneuver, 6 – cystic plate, 7 – umbilical groove (Image from personal collection of IN).

The common bile duct receives its vascular supply through small arteries coming from the right hepatic, superior posterior pancreaticoduodenal and gastro-duodenal arteries. Three areas of vascularization can be described for the extrahepatic biliary tree (Poston and Blumgart, 2003; Hann, 2012):

The hilar area: receives its blood supply from the right and left hepatic arteries. Which forms a rich network with the supraduodenal area.

The supraduodenal area: receives eight small arteries, with a diameter of 0.3 mm from the superior posterior pancreaticoduodenal artery, right hepatic artery, cystic artery and gastroduodenal artery. These small arteries usually give rise to two arcades, on the left (9 o'clock) and right (3 o'clock) flank of the common bile duct. 60% of arteries from this area run upwards from the inferior vessels, 38% run downward from the right hepatic artery and 2% are non-axial, emerging from the proper hepatic artery which has a parallel course with the common bile duct.

The retropancreatic area: receives its blood supply from the superior posterior pancreaticoduodenal artery.

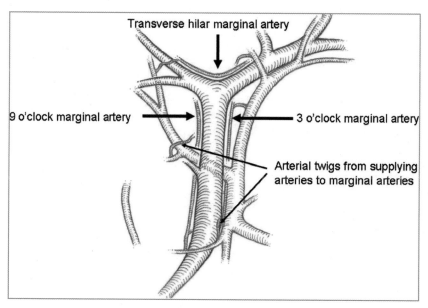

Figure 114. Blood supply to the bile ducts. Element 2: the marginal arteries. Marginal arteries are disposed at 3, 9 and, rarely, 12 o'clock (not shown) on the common bile duct/common hepatic duct. The hilar marginal artery runs across the top of the confluence of the right and left hepatic ducts [Figure reproduced with permission from John Wiley and Sons from Steven M. Strasberg, W. Scott Helton. An analytical review of vasculobiliary injury in laparoscopic and open cholecystectomy. HPB – The Official Journal of the International Hepato Pancreato Biliary Association. 13 (1), 1–14, 2011 (Strasberg and Helton, 2011)].

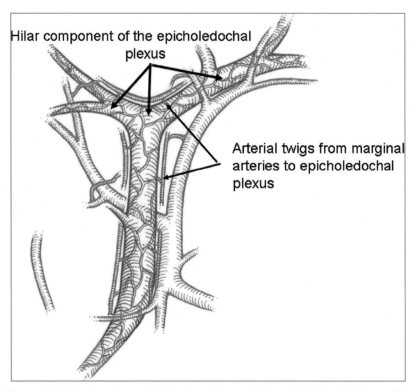

Figure 115. Blood supply to the bile ducts. Element 3: the epicholedochal plexus. The epicholedochal plexus is supplied by the marginal arteries and sometimes directly by the supplying arteries. The part of the network around the confluence of the right and left hepatic ducts has been termed the "hilar plexus". However, it is continuous with the plexus that surrounds the common duct and is probably best considered as the hilar component of the epicholedochal plexus [Figure reproduced with permission from John Wiley and Sons from Steven M. Strasberg, W. Scott Helton. An analytical review of vasculobiliary injury in laparoscopic and open cholecystectomy. HPB – The Official Journal of the International Hepato Pancreato Biliary Association. 13 (1), 1–14, 2011 (Strasberg and Helton, 2011)].

During hepatico-jejunostomy, the transection of the biliary duct should be above the insertion of the cystic duct, 1–2 cm below the confluence of the right and left hepatic ducts, to obtain an adequate blood supply of the upper cut margin.

VEINS

Rarely, there is a single cystic vein. Usually, the upper surface of the gallbladder drains through multiple small accessory portal veins directly into the liver, while the inferior surface drains through one of the two smaller veins.

LYPMHATICS

The gallbladder and extrahepatic biliary ducts drain into the lymph nodes located in the hepatoduodenal ligament.

INNERVATION

The extrahepatic biliary ducts receive their sympathetic and parasympathetic fibers through the hepatic plexus. The parasympathetic fibers originate from the hepatic branch of the anterior vagal trunk and from the celiac branch of the posterior vagal trunk. The sympathetic fibers originate from the celiac plexus. The celiac plexus sympathetic fibers come through the three splanchnic nerves. The gallbladder and liver receive also through the celiac plexus nervous fibers from the phrenic nerves, which explains pain radiation towards the right shoulder.

CHAPTER 20
HISTOLOGY

SORIN HOSTIUC, VALENTIN ENACHE

The gallbladder is a cavity organ whose wall consists of mucosa, muscularis and serosa. The mucosa includes simple cylindrical epithelium.

The gallbladder is a cavitary organ that contains:

A mucosal layer, containing high columnar cells, with a highly eosinophilic cytoplasm and, occasionally apical vacuoles. The nuclei are located basally, and are oval and uniform. Near the neck of the glands are present tubuloalveolar mucous glands, which are cuboid or low columnar, and have a clear or lightly basophilic cytoplasm (Mills, 2006).

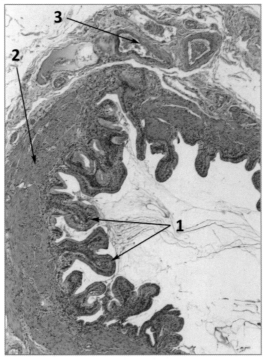

Figure 116. Hematoxylin and Eosin staining using 50x objective of normal gallbladder. 1 – mucosa, 2 – muscularis propria, 3 – blood vessels. It should be remembered that the gallbladder lacks submucosa (Image courtesy of VE, used with permission).

The lamina propria, contains loose connective tissue, nerve fibers, and vessels.

Muscle layer – contains bundles of fibers with various directions – circular, oblique or longitudinal, but which do not form well established layers as in other parts of the gastrointestinal system.

Subserosal layer – with a structure similar to the lamina propria; sometimes small aggregations of lymphocytes around the vessels, and paraganglia can be identified (Mills, 2006).

The gallblader does not have a muscularis mucosa nor a submucosal layer.

The extrahepatic bile ducts contain the following structures:

Mucosal layer – containing a single layer of high columnar cells, with basal nuclei.

A stromal layer, containing dense connective tissue with collagen and elastic fibers.

Duct of Wirsung contains an epithelial layer similar to that of the common bile duct, surrounded by a dense layer of connective tissue.

SECTION VIII – THE DUODENUM

Good surgical judgment comes from experience and experience comes from poor surgical judgment.

Chris Lillehei

CHAPTER 21

EMBRYOLOGY

RUXANDRA IRINA NEGOI

The embryological origin of the duodenum is from the primitive gut, at the boundary between the foregut and the midgut (Moore and Persaud, 2008). It initially has a C-shaped loop conformation, oriented with its convexity anteriorly, in the sagittal plane. During embryological development, the duodenal loop rotates, along with the stomach to the right. This process, is determined by the hepatocystic bud development into the layers of the ventral mesentery, will determine the fusion of the duodenum and pancreatic buds to the posterior abdominal wall, giving rise to the Treitz's coalescence fascia. Secondary to this process, the duodenum and the pancreas, except for the first part of the duodenum and the pancreatic tail, become secondary retroperitoneal organs (Negoi *et al.*, 2010). Since the foregut receives its vascular supply from the celiac artery and the midgut from the superior mesenteric artery, the duodenum has its vascularization from both sources (Sadler, 2009).

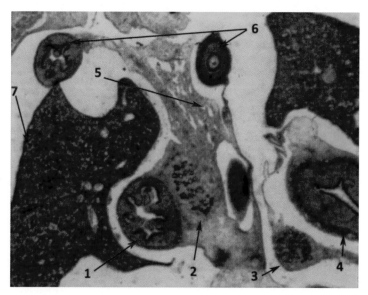

Figure 117. Transversal section through the upper abdomen of a rat embryo revealing the duodenum (1), the ventral pancreatic bud (2), the dorsal pancreatic bud (3), the stomach (4), the mesentery (5), the bowel loops (6), and the liver (7) (Figure courtesy of RIN).

CHAPTER 22

ANATOMY

IONUȚ NEGOI, MIRCEA BEURAN

The duodenum, the first segment of the small bowel, has its boundaries between the pyloric sphincter and Treitz's angle, at the duodenojejunal flexure. Its length is around 20–25 cm. On the posterior abdominal wall it projects between the first and fourth lumbar vertebrae. The duodenum has close anatomical relationships with the head and uncinate process of the pancreas, forming a common surgical entity. Except for the first 2.5 cm, which are located intraperitoneally, the duodenum and pancreas are secondary retroperitoneal organs, having the coalescence fascia of Treitz as an important surgical plane (Negoi *et al.*, 2010). On the anterior abdominal wall the duodenum projects onto the epigastric and mesogastric area.

TOPOGRAPHY

FIRST SEGMENT

The first duodenal segment is 5 cm long, extending from the pylorus to the upper duodenal flexure. Its initial intraperitoneal segment is located between the hepatoduodenal and gastrocolic peritoneum. Its projection on the posterior abdominal wall is to the right of the first lumbar vertebra.

SECOND SEGMENT

It is about 7.5 cm long, extends from the upper to lower duodenal flexures, and projects onto the right flank of the second and third lumbar vertebrae. The anterior surface of this duodenal segment its intersected by the transverse mesocolon.

THIRD SEGMENT

It is about 10 cm long and extends from the lower duodenal flexure to the left flank of the aorta and the mesentery root. Its posterior projection is onto the third and fourth lumbar vertebrae.

FOURTH SEGMENT

It is about 2.5 cm long and extends from the left aortic flank and the mesentery root until the duodenojejunal angle of Treitz. The projection of the fourth duodenal segment is onto the left flank of the second and third lumbar vertebrae. The duodenojejunal angle of Treitz, projects onto the left flank of the second lumbar vertebra, and is suspended from the right diaphragmatic pillar by the Treitz ligament, an embryological remnant of the primitive dorsal mesentery.

ANATOMICAL RELATIONSHIPS

FIRST SEGMENT

Anteriorly: Segment 4b of the liver, body of the gallbladder.
Posteriorly: Anterior to the coalescence fascia of Treitz – common bile duct, portal vein and gastroduodenal artery. Posterior to the coalescence fascia of Treitz – inferior vena cava.
Superiorly: Delimits the omental orifice of Winslow.
Inferiorly: Head of the pancreas

SECOND SEGMENT

Anteriorly – intersected by the root of the transverse mesocolon. Superior to the transverse mesocolon it has anatomical relationships with the fundus of the gallbladder and the right hemiliver. Inferior to the mesocolic root it has an anatomical relationship with the small bowel loops.

Posteriorly, deep to Treitz's coalescence fascia, it has anatomical relationships with the right kidney, right adrenal gland and the right renal pedicle (its most anterior structure being the renal vein).

Laterally, to the right: the ascending colon and the right colic angle (Negoi *et al.*, 2010).

THIRD SEGMENT

Anteriorly: the superior mesenteric vein and artery, the middle colic artery, the root of the mesentery and the small bowel loops.

Posteriorly, deep to the Treitz's coalescence fascia: the right ureter, right genital vessels, inferior vena cava, abdominal aorta.

Superiorly: the head and uncinate process of the pancreas, inferior pancreaticoduodenal artery. Also superiorly, but deep to Treitz's fascia is located the left renal vein. In the case of compression of the third segment of the duodenum, between the superior mesenteric artery, located anteriorly and the aorta, located posteriorly, a clinical picture of upper intestinal obstruction may occur.

FOURTH SEGMENT

Anteriorly: the small bowel loops, the transverse mesocolon and the posterior gastric surface.

Medially: the pancreatic head and superior mesenteric vessels.

Laterally: left ureter, medial surface of the left kidney, and the vascular arch of Treitz (inferior mesenteric vein and ascending branch of left colic artery).

Posteriorly: left gonadal vessels and left sympathetic chain, located on the left psoas muscle (Negoi *et al.*, 2010).

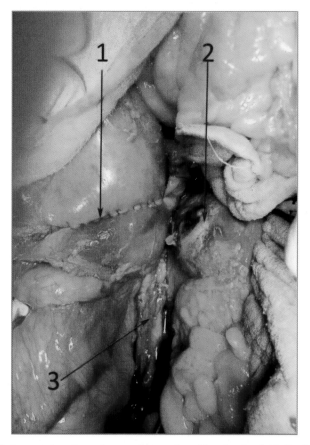

Figure 118. Intraoperative view of an aortic aneurism (2) – duodenal (1) fistula repaired by a double layer continuous suture of the duodenum and patch repair of the aortic aneurism.
3 – inferior mesenteric vein (Image courtesy of IN).

VASCULAR SUPPLY

ARTERIES

The first and fourth duodenal segments take their vascular supply from small arteries branching off from neighboring arteries. The first duodenal segment arteries branch off from the right gastric, gastroduodenal, supraduodenal and superior posterior pancreaticoduodenal arteries. The fourth duodenal segment is vascularized by the inferior pancreaticoduodenal artery and the first jejunal artery. The second and third duodenal segments have a common vascular supply with the pancreatic head, as detailed in that section of the book.

VEINS

They are homonymous to the corresponding arteries and drain into the portal vein.

LYMPHATICS

The duodenum has an important lymphatic network, which finally drains into the anterior and posterior pancreaticoduodenal lymph nodes.

INERVATION

The duodenum receives parasympathetic and sympathetic innervation from the celiac plexus. Parasympathetic fibers have their origin in the vagus nerve. Sympathetic fibers come from the greater and lesser splanchnic nerves (Negoi *et al.*, 2010).

ANATOMICAL SPACES AROUND THE DUODENUM

Peritoneal reflections from the duodenum to the neighboring organs give rise to anatomical spaces, which may be explained by the embryological development, with rotation and coalescence of the duodenum to the retroperitoneal space (Skandalakis *et al.*, 2004). The superior fossa of Treitz, found with an incidence of 30–50%, is determined by the inferior mesenteric vein, which presents an opening oriented caudally. The inferior duodenal fossa of Treitz is the most constant (50–75%) and opens cranially. The retroduodenal recess is located posterior to the fourth duodenal segment and has its opening to the left. These recesses may give rise to internal hernias.

CHAPTER 23
HISTOLOGY

SORIN HOSTIUC, VALENTIN ENACHE

The small intestine follows the same organization of the digestive tract, with four layers: mucosa, submucosa, muscularis propria and serosa. The mucosa and submucosa have folds, giving rise to the valves of Kerckring. The luminal surface of the mucosal epithelium presents intestinal villi, with a length ranging from 0.5–1.5 mm. The mucosal epithelium is composed of one-layer of cylindrical type cells and dispersed goblet cells. The goblet cells are rare in the duodenum, becoming more dense in the ileum. Between the epithelial villi there may be found invaginations of the intestinal glands, which are parallel and aligned along the basement membrane. Enterocytes from the villi and glands' structure are cylindrical cells, with a long axis perpendicular to the basement membrane. The lamina propria consists of loose connective tissue, vessels and nerves found just below the mucosal epithelial layer. The muscularis mucosa, is the deep layer of the mucosa, located just above the submucosa. The submucosa includes conjunctive tissue and a rich vascular and nervous network. The muscularis propria is well represented, and consists of two smooth muscle layers involved in gastrointestinal motility. The serosa consists of connective tissue covered by a flattened single-layer of epithelium (mesothelium) (Negoi *et al.*, 2010).

Malignant tumors of the duodenum are extremely rare, counting for 0.3% of all gastrointestinal tract tumors, but up to half of small bowel cancers (Fagniez & Rotman, 2001). A review of the Emergency Hospital of Bucharest experience regarding small bowel tumors revealed 57 cases during a time interval of 15 years (Negoi *et al.*, 2015c). 10 (17.5%) were duodenal tumors, 21 (36.8%) jejunum and 26 (45.6%) ileum tumors. Correlated with the bowel mean length, we have observed a higher prevalence for the adenocarcinoma (14.55 time higher) and for gastrointestinal stromal tumors (1.818 times higher) into the duodenum, when compared with the jejunum and ileum.

Bourgouin *et al.* looked for predictive factors of severe complications following pancreaticoduodenectomy for ampullary, bile duct and duodenal cancers (Bourgouin *et al.*, 2015). Multivariate analysis of this 10-year multicentre series revealed that only the external transanastomotic stents significantly decrease the morbidity (Hazard Ration = 0.37, 95% CI = 0.16–0.83, p = 0.016) and mortality (Hazard Ration = 0.12, 95% CI = 0.02–0.69, p = 0.017) (Bourgouin *et al.*, 2015).

SECTION IX – THE PANCREAS

The superior man is modest in his speech,
but exceeds in his actions.

Confucius (551 BC – 479 BC)

CHAPTER 24

EMBRYOLOGY

RUXANDRA IRINA NEGOI

Development of the pancreas begins in the fourth week of intrauterine life, from the ventral and dorsal pancreatic buds (Negoi *et al.*, 2010). These buds have their embryological origin in the duodenal loop endoderm. The ventral pancreatic bud evolves next to the origin of the hepatocystic bud, in the ventral mesentery. Initially, it has a bilobar conformation, with secondary atrophy of the left lobe.

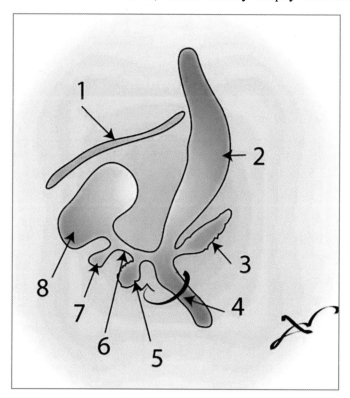

Figure 119. Schematic representation of the ventral pancreatic bud (5), dorsal pancreatic bud (3) and hepatocystic bud. 1 – septum transversum, 2 – stomach, 4 – duodenal loop, 6 – primordium of the common bile duct, 7 – primordium of the gallbladder, 8 – primordial of the liver (Personal courtesy RIN).

The dorsal pancreatic bud develops into the dorsal mesentery, cranially from the ventral pancreatic bud. Secondary to the clockwise rotation of the stomach and duodenal loop, with unequal growth of duodenal circumference, the ventral pancreatic bud rotates to the right, lying immediately posterior and inferior to the dorsal pancreatic bud (Sadler, 2009). At the end of this process, the ventral pancreatic bud fuses with the caudal surface of the dorsal bud. The pancreatic head and uncinate process originate in the ventral pancreatic bud. The rest of the pancreas has its embryological origin in the dorsal pancreatic bud (Moore and Persaud, 2008). A malformation of the rotational process of the two pancreatic buds may generate an annular pancreas, a ring of pancreatic tissue which surrounds the descending duodenum.

Each of the pancreatic buds has an embryological excretory duct. After the ducts' fusion, the two excretory ducts will anastomose. The main pancreatic duct of Wirsung has its embryological origin in the duct of the ventral pancreatic bud, the area of anastomosis and the distal segment of the dorsal duct. The accessory duct of Santorini has its origin in the proximal part of the dorsal bud's duct. In 10% of cases the ducts of the two pancreatic buds fail to fuse, giving rise to pancreas divisum (Sadler, 2009). The glandular anatomical structures of the pancreas have an endodermal origin. The endocrine islets of Langerhans have their origin in the neural crests.

The epithelial to mesenchymal transition (EMT) represents a key step during physiologic embryogenesis, with major impact on endodermic transformations, gastrulation and organ development, such as the peripheral nervous system, neural crest, heart, musculoskeletal and craniofacial structure (Beuran et al., 2015).

Table 12

Classification of EMT according to the biological context [Reprinted from Pancreatology, vol 15 (3), Mircea Beuran, Ionut Negoi, Sorin Paun, Adriana Daniela Ion, Coralia Bleotu, Ruxandra Irina Negoi, Sorin Hostiuc, The epithelial to mesenchymal transition in pancreatic cancer: A systematic review, pages no. 217–225, Copyright (2015), with permission from Elsevier (Beuran et al., 2015)]

Characteristics	Types of EMT		
	Type 1	Type 2	Type 3
Moment of appearance during human life	Embryo formation: • Organ development	Adult life: • Trauma • Inflammation	Adult life: • Epithelial cancer
Physiological processes in which EMT is involved	Generates the first set of mesenchymal cells = primary mesenchyme	Wound healing Tissue regeneration Organ fibrosis	
Pathological processes in which EMT is involved	Without	Ongoing fibrosis with organ destruction	Systemic progression = Metastases

Secondary to this process, the epithelial cells, usually stuck to the basement membrane, acquire a high mobility and migratory capacity. Once the organ development is complete, these cells become differentiated, losing their mesenchymal phenotype. In a review by our group, we detailed the "…essential role in the local progression and metastasis of pancreatic cancer. Areas of interest are the cross-linking between cells undergoing EMT and pancreatic cancer stem cells, and the correlation between EMT and chemoresistance to standard therapies".

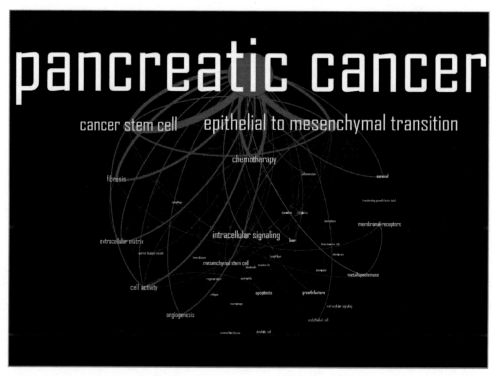

Figure 120. Correlation between pancreatic cancer, cancer stem cells and epithelial mesenchymal transition (This graph is from personal courtesy of IN. The semantic analysis was performed on the most cited 100 articles from Scopus Elsevier database regarding epithelial to mesenchymal transition in pancreatic cancer).

During carcinogenesis, malignant pancreatic cells at the primary site acquire the ability to undergo EMT, a transformation associated with increased mobility. The reverse process at secondary sites, mesenchymal to epithelial transition (MET), has devastating consequences, allowing neoplastic epithelial cells to invade surrounding tissues and spread to distant sites. The consequences of EMT are the loss of E-cadherin expression and the acquisition of mesenchymal markers including fibronectin or vimentin. Detailed knowledge of the molecular processes underlying EMT has opened up the possibilities for new therapeutic agents. These include an EMT approach for patients with early cancers, to prevent invasion and dissemination, and anti-MET therapy for patients with established metastasis." We concluded that: "The current literature shows a strong correlation between EMT and the systemic aggressiveness of pancreatic tumors. Individualized therapy, targeting the process of EMT and its cross-linking with cancer stem cells, may increase the survival of patients with pancreatic cancer." [Reprinted from Pancreatology, vol. 15 (3), Mircea Beuran, Ionut Negoi, Sorin Paun, Adriana Daniela Ion, Coralia Bleotu, Ruxandra Irina Negoi, Sorin Hostiuc, The epithelial to mesenchymal transition in pancreatic cancer: A systematic review, pp. 217–225, Copyright (2015), with permission from Elsevier (Beuran *et al.*, 2015)].

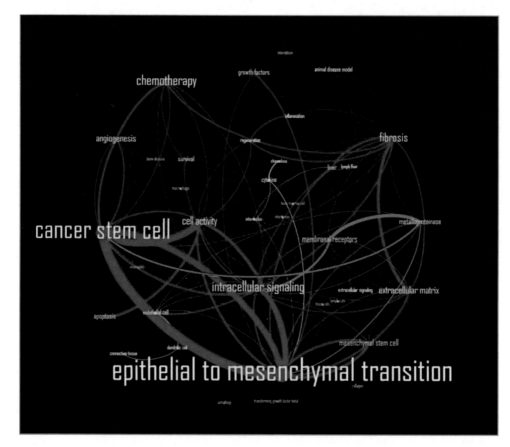

Figure 121. Correlation between resistance to chemotherapy, cancer stem cells and epithelial mesenchymal transition in pancreatic cancer (This graph is from personal courtesy of IN. The semantic analysis was performed on the most cited 100 articles from Scopus Elsevier database regarding epithelial to mesenchymal transition in pancreatic cancer).

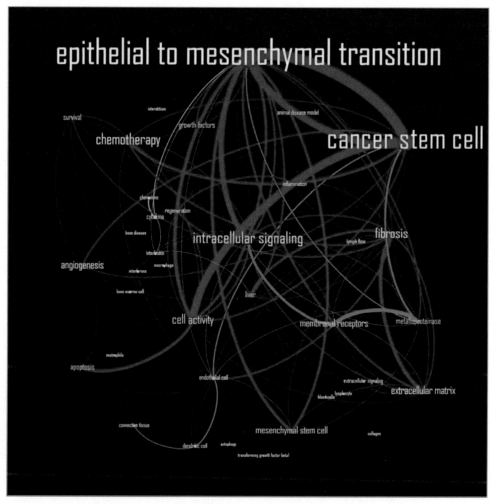

Figure 122. Correlation between resistance to chemotherapy, cancer stem cells and epithelial mesenchymal transition in pancreatic cancer. (This graph is from personal courtesy of IN. The semantic analysis was performed on the most cited 100 articles from Scopus Elsevier database regarding epithelial to mesenchymal transition in pancreatic cancer).

CHAPTER 25
ANATOMY

IONUȚ NEGOI, MIRCEA BEURAN

EXTERNAL CONFORMATION

The pancreas is a digestive gland, with a mixed exocrine (pancreatic juice produced by glandular acini) and endocrine (hormones secreted by islets of Langerhans) function. It has a weight of about 70–90 grams and a length of about 15–18 cm (Negoi *et al.*, 2010). The classical anatomy description for the pancreas, a head, body and tail. The surgical anatomy also describes a neck and an uncinate process.

The head has a circular shape, with anterior and posterior surfaces, and a circumference in close relationship with the duodenum. Inferiorly and to the left, the uncinate process continues with the pancreatic head. The pancreatic neck is about 2 to 3 cm in length, at the boundary between the head and body. It is defined as the pancreatic segment located anterior to the portal and the superior mesenteric vein. The body has a prismatic shape and continues with the tail, located in the splenic hilum.

TOPOGRAPHY

Except for its tail, the pancreas is a secondary retroperitoneal organ, presenting posteriorly the coalescence fascia of Treitz. On the anterior abdominal wall, the pancreas is projected onto the periumbilical and left upper quadrant. The posterior projection is at the level of the first to third lumbar vertebrae.

ANATOMICAL RELATIONSHIPS

PANCREATIC HEAD

The pancreatic head is traversed on its anterior surface by the transverse mesocolon root. Above the transverse mesocolon, it has anatomical relationships with the pyloric area of the stomach. Below the transverse mesocolon, the pancreatic head has anatomical relationships with the small bowel loops and the middle colic artery. On the anterior surface of the pancreatic head is located the anterior pancreaticoduodenal vascular arcade.

Posteriorly, between the pancreas and Treitz's fascia may be found the portal vein, common bile duct and the posterior pancreaticoduodenal vascular arcade.

Posterior to Treitz's fascia, the pancreatic head has anatomical relationships with the right kidney, the renal pedicle (the most anterior element being the right renal vein), the inferior vena cava and the right genital vessels.

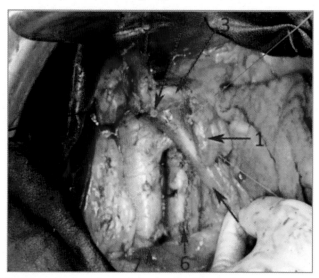

Figure 123. Intraoperative view of the interaorticocaval lymphadenectomy during pancreaticoduodenectomy: 1 – pancreatic stump, 2 – superior mesenteric vein, 3 – common hepatic artery, 4 – gastroduodenal artery stump, 5 – proper hepatic artery, 6 – aorta, 7 – inferior vena cava (Image courtesy of MB).

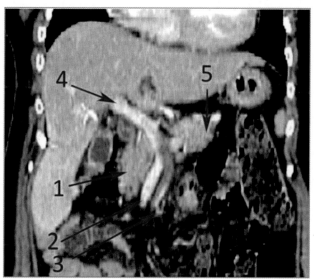

Figure 124. Computed Tomography, coronal section, revealing the pancreatic head (1), the superior mesenteric vein (2) and artery (3), portal vein (4) and the pancreatic body (5) (Image courtesy of Radiology and Imagistics Department, Emergency Hospital of Bucharest).

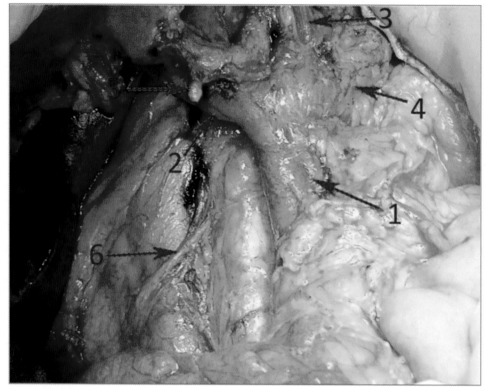

Figure 125. Intraoperative view of the site of resection during pancreatico-duodenectomy: 1 – superior mesenteric vein, 2 – portal vein, 3 – left gastric vein draining into the splenic vein (4). 5 – gastroduodenal artery stump, 6 – right genital artery (Image courtesy of MB).

UNCINATE PROCESS

The uncinate process has great variability in its length, but generally has the following anatomical relationships:
Superiorly: the left renal vein.
Inferiorly: the third duodenal segment.
Anteriorly: superior mesenteric vessels.

BODY

The anterior surface of the body has an anatomical relationship, via the omental bursa with the posterior surface of the stomach. Its inferior surface, located below the transverse mesocolon, has anatomical relationships with the duo-denojejunal angle of Treitz and the small bowel loops.

Posteriorly, between the pancreas and Treitz's fascia are located the splenic vessels. The splenic artery has a sinuous trajectory near the upper margin of the pancreatic body. The splenic vein has a linear course, in close contact with the posterior surface of the pancreatic body. Posterior to Treitz's fascia, the pancreatic body has relationships with the aorta, the origin of the superior mesenteric artery, the left renal vein, the left adrenal gland and the left kidney.

TAIL

The pancreatic tail is its only intraperitoneal segment, located in the splenorenal peritoneal ligament, in close contact with the splenic hilum. In this area, the splenic vessels are located anterior to the pancreatic tail.

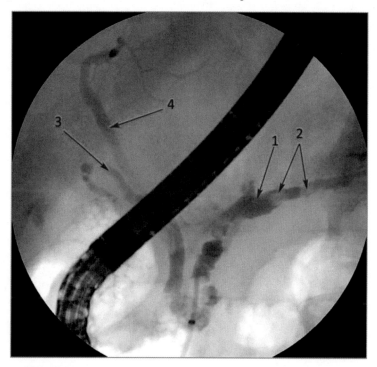

Figure 126. Endoscopic Retrograde Cholangiopancreatography revealing a dilated pancreatic duct (1) with stones (2). Also can be observed, the cystic duct (3) which joins the common hepatic duct (4) in a parallel fashion (Image courtesy of Gastroenterology Department, Emergency Hospital of Bucharest).

Table 13
Distribution of pancreatic parenchyma according to usual surgical resections
[Adapted after (Kooby *et al.*, 2011)]

Anatomical landmarks	Distribution of pancreatic parenchyma
To the left on the superior mesenteric – portal vein	60–70% of pancreatic parenchyma
Typical Whipple resection	Resection of 35% of pancreatic parenchyma
Endocrine and exocrine insufficiency – Resection of > 80% of pancreatic parenchyma.	

VASCULAR SUPPLY

ARTERIES

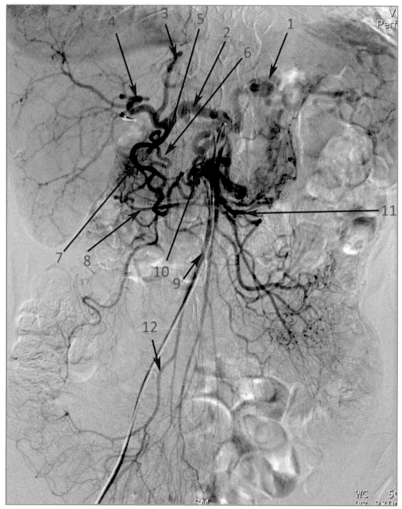

Figure 127. Angiography of the superior mesenteric artery (9) with significant retrograde flow of the hepatic and splenic vascularization, suggesting celiac trunk stenosis. This arterial conformation is especially dangerous during pancreaticoduo-denectomy, transection of the gastroduodenal artery causing significant liver ischemia. A trial clamping of the gastroduodenal artery with evaluation of the proper hepatic artery arterial flow is mandatory to prevent an ominous prognosis: 1 – splenic artery, 2 – common hepatic artery , 3 – left hepatic artery, 4 – right hepatic artery, 5 – gastro-duodenal artery, 6 – superior posterior pancreaticoduodenal artery, 7 – superior anterior pancreaticoduodenal artery, 8 – right gastroepiploic artery, 9 – superior mesenteric artery, 10 – inferior pancreaticoduodenal artery, 11 – first jejunal artery, 12 ileocolic artery (Figure courtesy of Emergency Hospital of Bucharest, Department of Angiography).

PANCREATIC HEAD

The pancreatic head has a common vascular supply with the second and third segments of the duodenum, represented by the anterior and posterior pancreaticoduodenal vascular arcades.

The anterior pancreaticoduodenal vascular arcade is formed by the superior anterior pancreaticoduodenal artery (terminal branch of the gastroduodenal artery) which anastomoses with the anterior branch of the inferior pancreaticoduodenal artery (branch of the superior mesenteric artery). The posterior pancreaticoduodenal artery is formed by the superior posterior pancreaticoduodenal artery (collateral branch of the gastroduodenal artery) which anastomoses with the posterior branch of the inferior pancreaticoduodenal artery. The superior posterior pancreaticoduodenal artery has its origin posterior to the first duodenal segment, and has an initial trajectory anterior to the common bile duct, then encircles it, to pass downward posterior to it. From these two arcades will emerge terminal arteries for the duodenum and pancreatic head.

BODY AND TAIL

The pancreatic body and tail have an individual vascular supply, coming from the splenic artery through three sources: the dorsal pancreatic, great pancreatic and artery of the pancreatic tail. The dorsal pancreatic artery branches off the splenic artery close to its origin. After a short trajectory posterior to the pancreatic body it divides into three branches, two to the right and one to the left. The right branches will anastomose with the anterior and posterior pancreaticoduodenal arcades. The left branch is termed the inferior pancreatic artery, with a trajectory to the left, on the inferior margin of the pancreatic body.

The great pancreatic artery emerges from the splenic artery at the junction of the right third with the left two thirds. Posterior to the pancreatic body it will divide into three branches, which terminate in the inferior pancreatic artery. The pancreatic tail's artery emerges in the splenic hilum, usually from terminal branches of the splenic artery. It terminates, also in the inferior pancreatic artery.

THE SURGICAL ANATOMY OF THE INFERIOR
PANCREATICODUODENAL ARTERY

The inferior pancreaticoduodenal artery (IPDA) forms a common trunk with the first jejunal artery (FJA) or arises directly from the SMA, usually from its left dorsal aspect (Cho, Yamamoto and Kainuma, 2014). The IPDA is usually located at 38 ± 8.8 mm from the origin of the SMA (Kawai et al., 2008; Cho, Yamamoto and Kainuma, 2014). Analyzing imagistic data of 160 patients, Inoue et al. showed that 134 patients had a single IPDA, 25 had two IPDAs (termed anterior and posterior IPDAs) while IPDA lacked in one case (Inoue et al., 2015).

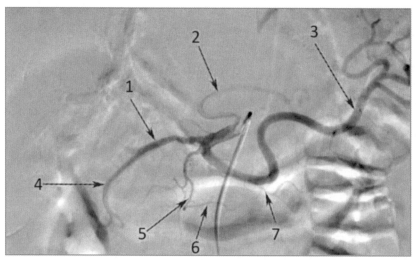

Figure 128. Angiography of the celiac artery revealing the common hepatic artery (1), left gastric artery (2), splenic artery (3), gastroduodenal artery (4), dorsal pancreatic artery (5) with its left branch termed the inferior pancreatic artery (6) and great pancreatic artery (7) (Figure courtesy of Emergency Hospital of Bucharest, Department of Angiography).

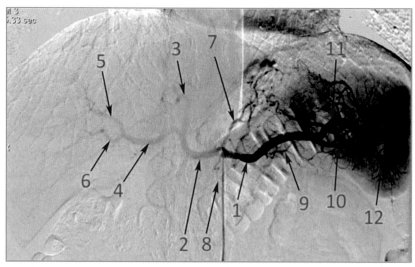

Figure 129. Angiography of the celiac artery revealing the splenic artery (1), common hepatic artery (2), left hepatic artery (3), right hepatic artery (4), right anterior sectional artery (5), right posterior sectional artery (6), left gastric artery (7), dorsal pancreatic artery (8), great pancreatic artery (9), inferior (10) and superior (11) lobar splenic branches and inferior segmental branch (12) (Figure from the courtesy of Emergency Hospital of Bucharest, Department of Angiography).

The IPDA emerged from a common trunk with the first jejunal artery in 71.6% of cases, independently from the SMA in 24.6% and from a replaced right hepatic artery in 3.8% of cases. Its origin was located on the dorsal aspect of the

SMA in 65.6% of patients, on the right aspect in 20.8% and on the left aspect in 13.7% of patients. The first jejunal vein runs posterior to the SMA in 67.5–83.3% of cases, two or more branches had an anterior and posterior course in 21.9% of cases and an anterior course in 10.6–16.7% of patients (Nakamura *et al.*, 2013; Inoue *et al.*, 2015).

REPLACED RIGHT HEPATIC ARTERY

During pancreaticoduodenectomy, mandatory early identification of the anatomic variants, such as replaced or accessory hepatic arteries originating in the SMA is necessary (Pallisera, Morales and Ramia, 2014).

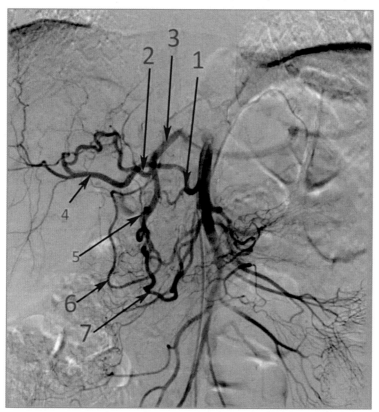

Figure 130. Angiography of the superior mesenteric artery revealing a replaced right hepatic artery (1 and 4) with the origin at this level, a left hepatic artery (2) with the origin into the common hepatic artery (3). 5 – gastroduodenal artery, 6 – posterior pancreaticoduodenal arcade, 7 – anterior pancreaticoduodenal arcade (Figure courtesy of Emergency Hospital of Bucharest, Department of Angiography).

The most common abnormalities of the hepatic vasculature include a replaced right hepatic artery (RHA) (11–21%), replaced LHA (3.8–10%), accessory RHA or LHA (0.8–8%) and celiac artery stenosis (2–7.6%) (Shukla *et al.*, 2010). Analyzing their 254 pancreatoduodenectomies, Yang *et al.* found that significant anatomical variations in the hepatic arterial system was encountered in as many as 20% of cases, including a common hepatic artery from the SMA (2.34%) and a replaced RHA from the SMA (9.82%) (Yang *et al.*, 2007).

VEINS

The pancreatic veins are similar to the corresponding arteries, and drain into the splenic, superior mesenteric or portal vein. The anatomy of the gastrocolic trunk of Henle was studied by Miyazawa *et al.* in 120 patients (Miyazawa *et al.*, 2015).

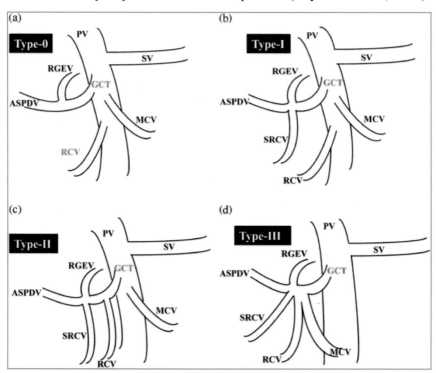

Figure 131. Anterior superior pancreaticoduodenal vein (ASPDV) and the types of tributaries of the GCT: (a) Type-0 was defined as a type where no superior right colic vein (SRCV), right colic vein (RCV) or middle colic vein (MCV) drained into the gastrocolic trunk (GCT). In Type-0 cases, the GCT was formed as a confluence of the anterior superior pancreatico-duodenal vein (ASPDV) and right gastroepiploic vein (RGEV). (b) Type-I was defined as a venous trunk of the tripod confluence consisting of the RGEV, ASPDV and SRCV. In Type-I cases, one colic drainage vein joined the GCT. (c) Type-II was defined as a venous trunk where the RCV or MCV additionally joined the Type-I GCT. In Type-II cases, two colic drainage veins joined the GCT. (d) Type-III was defined as a venous trunk where the SRCV, RCV and MCV drained into the GCT. In Type-III cases, three colic drainage veins joined the GCT [Figure reproduced with permission from John Wiley and Sons from Motoki Miyazawa, Manabu Kawai, Seiko Hirono, Ken-ichi Okada, Atsushi Shimizu, Yuji Kitahata, Hiroki Yamaue. Preoperative evaluation of the confluent drainage veins to the gastrocolic trunk of Henle: understanding the surgical vascular anatomy during pancreaticoduodenectomy. Journal of Hepato-Biliary-Pancreatic Sciences, 22 (5), 386–391, 2015 (Miyazawa *et al.*, 2015)].

They identified by three dimensional CT the gastrocolic trunk in 83.3% of cases: Type-0 in 7%, Type-I in 71%, Type-II in 20% and Type-III in 2% of patients (Miyazawa *et al.*, 2015).

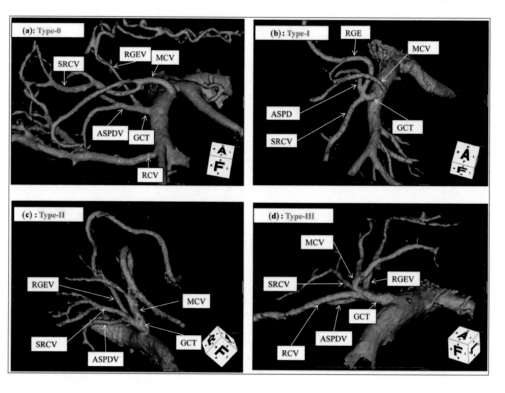

Figure 132. Representative cases of every type of variation of the gastrocolic trunk (GCT) detected by 3D multidetector-row computed tomography (MDCT). The frequencies of Type-0, Type-I, Type-II and Type-III were 7% (n=7), 71% (n=71), 20% (n=20) and 2% (n=2), respectively. (a) Type-0: the GCT was formed by only the confluence of the anterior superior pancreaticoduodenal vein (ASPDV) and right gastroepiploic vein (RGEV). (b) Type-I: the GCT was formed by the tripod confluence consisting of the RGEV, ASPDV and superior right colic vein (SRCV). The middle colic vein (MVC) drained cranially to the GCT. (c) Type-II: two colic drainage veins consisting of the SRCV and right colic vein (RCV) or MCV drained into the GCT. (d) Type-III: three colic drainage veins consisting of the SRCV, RCV and MCV drained into the GCT [Figure reproduced with permission from John Wiley and Sons from Motoki Miyazawa, Manabu Kawai, Seiko Hirono, Ken-ichi Okada, Atsushi Shimizu, Yuji Kitahata, Hiroki Yamaue. Preoperative evaluation of the confluent drainage veins to the gastrocolic trunk of Henle: understanding the surgical vascular anatomy during pancreaticoduodenectomy. Journal of Hepato-Biliary-Pancreatic Sciences, 22 (5), 386–391, 2015 (Miyazawa *et al.*, 2015)].

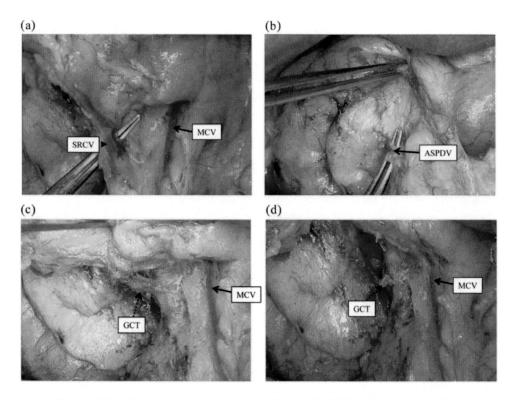

Figure 133. The approach to the gastrocolic trunk (GCT) during pancreatico-duodenectomy. (a) This case is Type-I. The middle colic vein (MVC) (arrow) directly drained into the superior mesenteric vein (SMV). The arrowhead shows the superior right colic vein (SRCV). First, the SRCV (arrowhead), which drained into the GCT, was divided. The arrow shows the MCV. (b) The arrow shows the anterior superior pancreaticoduodenal vein (ASPDV). Next, ASPDV was divided. (c) Then, the fat tissue around the lower side of the GCT was safely dissected. Finally, the neck of the GCT (dashed arrow) was identified following the division of the SRCV. (d) The surgical field was developed for tunneling between the anterior surface of the SMV and the pancreas after dissection of the GCT (dashed arrow). The MCV (arrow) was preserved. [Figure reproduced with permission from John Wiley and Sons from Motoki Miyazawa, Manabu Kawai, Seiko Hirono, Ken-ichi Okada, Atsushi Shimizu, Yuji Kitahata, Hiroki Yamaue. Preoperative evaluation of the confluent drainage veins to the gastrocolic trunk of Henle: understanding the surgical vascular anatomy during pancreaticoduodenectomy. Journal of Hepato-Biliary-Pancreatic Sciences, 22 (5), 386–391, 2015 (Miyazawa *et al.*, 2015)].

LYMPHATICS

The origin of the lymphatic drainage of the pancreas is in an abundant perilobular network. These small lobular channels coalesce to form several lymphatic channels, which drain into the regional lymph nodes, and from here further into the thoracic duct (Shoup and Smith, 2011). According to the embryological origin of the pancreas, from a ventral and dorsal pancreatic bud, the lymphatics may be divided into right sided and left sided flows:

- The right sided flow, which drains the derivatives of the ventral pancreatic bud: caudal segment of the head and uncinate process.

- The left sided flow, which drains the derivatives of the dorsal pancreatic bud: upper segment of the head, neck, body and tail.

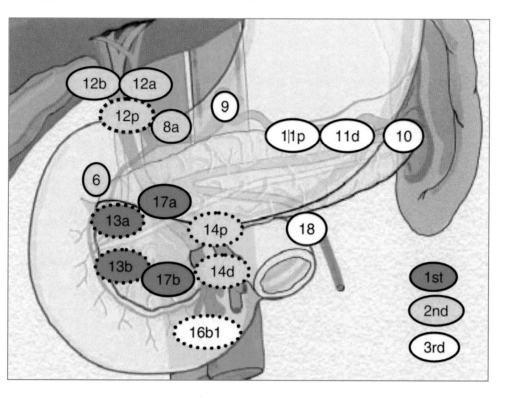

Figure 134. Japanese Pancreas Society lymph node groups; first-, second- and third-order lymph node groups are shown. Dotted lines indicate posteriorly positioned lymph node stations [Figure reproduced with permission from John Wiley and Sons from N. Alexakis, C. Halloran, M. Raraty, P. Ghaneh, R. Sutton, J.P. Neoptolemos. British Journal of Surgery. 91 (11), 1410–1427, 2004. (Alexakis *et al.*, 2004)].

Lymph nodes	Carcinoma of the head of the pancreas ($n = 90$)	Carcinoma of the distal bile duct ($n = 22$)	Carcinoma of the papilla of Vater ($n = 27$)
1	0	0	0
2	0	0	0
3	0	0	0
4	0	0	1 (4)
5	0	0	0
6	13 (14)	0	0
7	0	0	0
8	12 (13)	1 (4)	0
9	2 (2)	1 (4)	0
10	1 (1)	0	0
11	16 (18)	0	0
12	17 (19)	5 (23)	1 (4)
13	46 (51)	3 (14)	11 (41)
14	21 (23)	2 (9)	3 (11)
15	0	0	0
16	23 (26)	2 (9)	0
17	35 (39)	1 (4)	6 (22)
18	3 (3)	1 (4)	0

Values in parentheses represent percentages

Figure 135. Lymph node involvement in patients with carcinoma of the head of the pancreas region. Nomenclature of perigastric lymph nodes in patients with carcinoma of the head of the pancreas and lymph nodes in carcinoma of the head of the pancreas region: 1. right cardiac lymph nodes; 2. left cardiac lymph nodes; 3. lesser curvature lymph nodes; 4. greater curvature lymph nodes; 5. suprapyloric lymph nodes; 6. infrapyloric lymph nodes; 7. lymph nodes around the left gastric artery; 8. lymph nodes around the common hepatic artery; 9. lymph nodes around the coeliac trunk; 10. lymph nodes at the hilus of the spleen; 11. lymph nodes along the splenic artery; 12. lymph nodes of the hepatoduodenal ligament; 13. posterior pancreaticoduodenal lymph nodes; 14. lymph nodes around the superior mesenteric artery; 15. lymph nodes along the middle colic artery; 16. para-aortic lymph nodes; 17. anterior pancreaticoduodenal lymph nodes; 18. inferior pancreatic body lymph nodes [Table reproduced with permission from John Wiley and Sons, from A. Nakao, A. Harada, T. Nonami, T. Kaneko, H. Murakami, S. Inoue, Y. Takeuchi, H. Takagi. Lymph node metastases in carcinoma of the head of the pancreas region. British Journal of Surgery, 82, 399–402, 1995. (Nakao *et al.*, 1995)].

INNERVATION

The pancreas has parasympathetic and sympathetic innervation coming from the celiac plexus. The parasympathetic fibers have their origin in the posterior vagal trunk. The sympathetic fibers come from the greater, smaller and least splanchnic nerves. In an attempt to decrease the pain intensity in unresectable pancreatic tumors, the sensitive fibers can be interrupted, through celiac plexus or splanchnic nerves neurolysis.

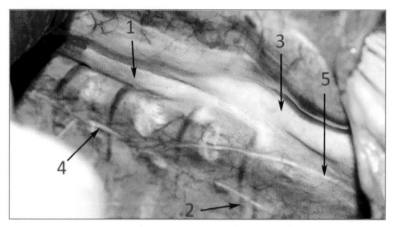

Figure 136. Dissection on a cadaveric model revealing the azygos vein (1), the posterior intercostal veins (2), aorta (3), thoracic sympathetic chain (4) and greater splanchnic nerve (5) (Image from personal courtesy of SH, IN).

According to the Japanese General Rules for the Study of Pancreatic Cancer, the nerve plexuses of the pancreatic head are (Japan Pancreas Society, 2003):

• Pancreatic head plexus I (PL ph I) is represented by the nervous bundle that connects the right celiac ganglion (PL ce – celiac plexus) with the pancreatic head.

• Pancreatic head plexus II (PL ph II) is represented by the nervous bundle that connects the SMA right hemi-circumference (PL sma – superior mesenteric artery plexus) with the pancreatic head.

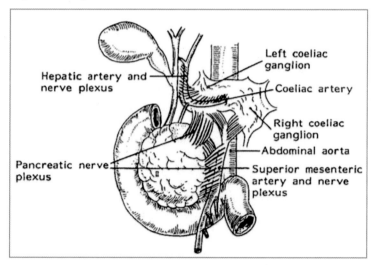

Figure 137. Nerves for the pancreatic head [Figure reproduced with permission from John Wiley and Sons, from T. Nagakawa, K. Mori, T. Nakano, M. Kadoya, H. Kobayashi, T. Akiyama, M. Kayahara, T. Ohta, K. Ueno, Y. Higashino, I. Konishi, I. Miyazaki. Perineural invasion of carcinoma of the pancreas and biliary tract. British Journal of Surgery. 80, 619–621, 1993 (Nagakawa *et al.*, 1993)].

From the nervous celiac plexus emerges to the left, the splenic plexus (PL sp), which surrounds the splenic artery, and to the right, the common hepatic artery plexus (PL cha). The PL cha is continued by the nervous plexus within the hepato-duodenal ligament (PL hdl) (Kondo, 2010).

MESOPANCREAS

The mesopancreas is represented by the retropancreatic retroportal tissue, on the right side of the SMA and celiac artery, through which runs, the inferior pancreaticoduodenal arteries and veins, lymphatics and nerve plexus (Adham and Singhirunnusorn, 2012). Adham and Singhirunnusorn characterized an inverted triangle, "the mesopancreas triangle", with the base lying on the posterior surface of the SMV and PV, the summit lying on the anterior surface of the aorta between the celial trunk (CT) and SMA origin, and limited on each side by the right semi-circumferences of the CT and SMA plexus (Adham and Singhirunnusorn, 2012).

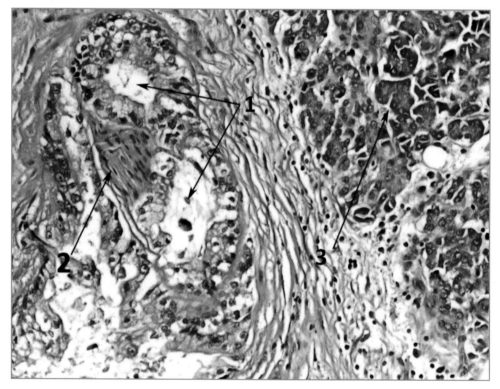

Figure 138. Hematoxylin and Eosin staining using 200 × objective of pancreatic ductal adenocarcinoma (1) with perineurial invasion (2). 3 – normal aspect of exocrine pancreatic tissue (Image courtesy of VE, used with permission).

Although it is not surrounded by a fibrous sheath or fascia, the mesopancreas should be accepted as a "mesentery" of the head of the pancreas (Agrawal *et al.*, 2010). The importance of this anatomical entity comes from the fact that it is the most frequent site of R1 resection (Gaedcke *et al.*, 2010). The goal of total mesopancreas excision should be differentiated from the extended lympha-denectomy (Peparini and Chirletti, 2013). Skeletonization of the right side of the SMA and CT at their origin and between them on the anterior surface of the aorta, considered to be fundamental steps in total mesopancreas excision, will remove all the neurolymphovascular and soft tissue, achieving partial lymphadenectomy of the interaortocaval and preaortic areas (Peparini and Chirletti, 2012). The optimal dissection and skeletonization of the SMA can be achieved with Harmonic scalpel or LigaSure devices, knowing that division of the soft tissue adjacent to the SMA with a stapler or a clamp and cut technique may leave up to 43% of the meso-pancreas in situ, with an increased risk of an R1 resection (Evans and Pisters, 2003; Baque *et al.*, 2009). Analysis of 6 patients who had pancreatic head carcinoma invading the SMV showed that the nerve plexus covering the SMA was involved in 4 cases, mainly behind the SMA and reaching as far as the left side of the SMA in 3 cases (Noto *et al.*, 2005).

CHAPTER 26

HISTOLOGY

VALENTIN ENACHE, SORIN HOSTIUC

The pancreas is a mixed gland, with both endocrine and exocrine function. The microscopical unit of the pancreas is called the lobule. Each lobule contains acini, ducts, and islets of Langerhans, and is separated from the neighboring lobules through intralobular connective tissue in which are identifiable vessels and nerve fibers.

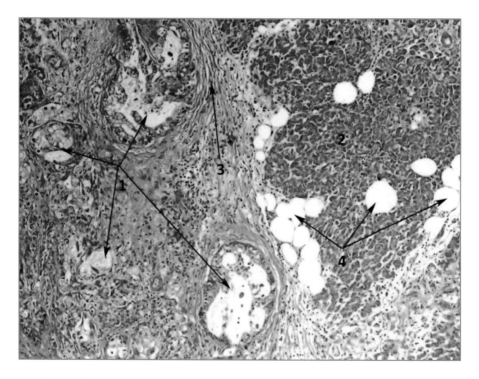

Figure 139. Hematoxylin and Eosin staining using 40 × objective of pancreatic ductal adenocarcinoma (1). 2 – normal aspect of pancreatic acini, 3 – desmoplastic reaction surrounding pancreatic adenocarcinoma, 4 – adipocytes (Image courtesy of VE, used with permission).

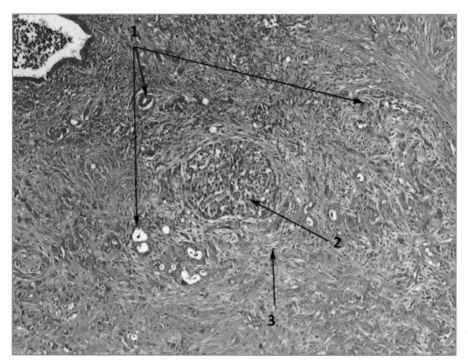

Figure 140. Hematoxylin and Eosin staining using 40 × objective of pancreatic ductal adenocarcinoma (1). 2 – normal aspect of islet of Langerhans, 3 – desmoplastic reaction surrounding pancreatic adenocarcinoma (Image courtesy of VE, used with permission).

The acini are the exocrine, secretory mass of the pancreas, and consists of a single layer of polygonal cells surrounding a central lumen. Acinar cells are intensely polar, with a basophilic base at which level the nucleus is identifiable, and an apical part containing an intense eosinophilic cytoplasm rich in zymogen granules (Hruban, Pitman and Klimstra, 2007). The ducts represent a transport system that transports the exocrine secretion from the acini to the duodenum. They start at the acinar level, where they consists of a layer of flat or cuboidal cells. These lumens unite into intercalated ducts, with an epithelial layer consisting of flat/cuboid cells. Both acinar and intercalated ducts lack a significant connective, surrounding tissue. The next division is represented by interlobular ducts, which have a dense connective tissue surrounding the luminal layer. The main pancreatic ducts have a flat epithelium surrounded by a thick connective tissue containing periductal ductules and smooth muscle fibers (Hruban, Pitman and Klimstra, 2007). The acinar cells, which are the predominant cells within the exocrine lobule, are pyramidal in shape. The pancreatic ducts are lined by epithelial cells: flat for the intralobular ducts, pyramidal cells for the interlobular ducts and columnar cells interspersed with goblet cells for the main pancreatic duct (Hartley and Finch-Jones, 2003).

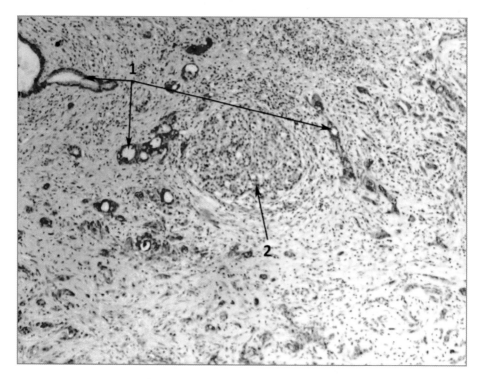

Figure 141. Immunohistochemistry expression of cytokeratin 7, using 40 × objective. Pancreatic ducats adenocarcinoma cells (1) showing immunoreactivity, while islets of Langerhans tissue shows the absence of reactivity (2) (Image courtesy of VE, used with permission).

The islets of Langerhans have a diameter of 100–200 μm, and include the following cellular populations: (a) alpha, producing glucagon, (b) beta, secreting insulin, (c) delta, secreting somatostatin and (d) PP cells, producing pancreatic polypeptide, and (e) epsilon, producing ghrelin. There are two main subtypes of islets: most are compact, well circumscribed, identified usually in the body or tail of the gland; a small number (around 10%) are diffuse, usually located in the posteroinferior part of the head (Mills 2006). These islets represents only 2% of the pancreatic weight, but receive up to 20% of the pancreatic vascular flow (Hartley and Finch-Jones, 2003).

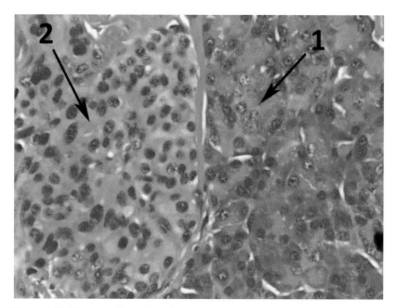

Figure 142. Hematoxylin and Eosin staining using 200 × objective of pancreatic
neuroendocrine tumors (NET G1) (2), 1 – normal aspect of exocrine pancreatic tissue
(Image courtesy of VE, used with permission).

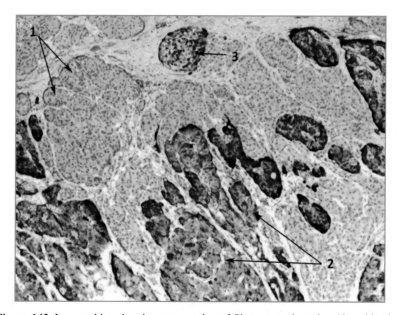

Figure 143. Immunohistochemistry expression of Chromogranin, using 40 × objective.
Pancreatic neuroendocrine tumor cells (2) and normal islet of Langerhans (3) showing
immunoreactivity, while exocrine pancreatic tissue shows the absence of reactivity (1)
(Image courtesy of VE, used with permission).

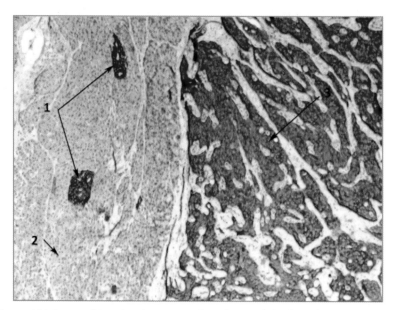

Figure 144. Immunohistochemistry expression of synaptophysin, using 40 × objective. Pancreatic neuroendocrine tumor cells (3) and normal islet of Langerhans (1) showing immunoreactivity, while exocrine pancreatic tissue shows the absence of reactivity (2) (Image courtesy of VE, used with permission).

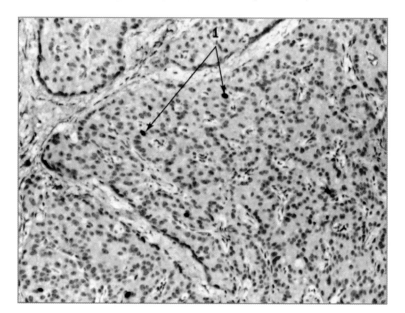

Figure 145. Immunohistochemistry expression of Ki67, using 100 × objective. Pancreatic neuroendocrine tumor cells showing immunoreactivity (1) in less than 2% of cells, correlating with a NET G1 tumor (Image courtesy of VE, used with permission).

CHAPTER 27

PANCREATIC CANCER

IONUȚ NEGOI, MIRCEA BEURAN, ALEXANDRU RUNCANU

RESECTION MARGIN

According to NCCN guidelines the survival benefits of an R1 resection may be comparable to definitive chemoradiation without surgery (NCCN Clinical Practice Guidelines in Oncology, 2015). On the other hand, according to Konstantinidis *et al*, the surgical procedures with microscopic tumor at the resection margin may have improved survival compared with locally advanced unresectable pancreatic cancers. In their study, R0 resections had a survival benefit compared with R1 resections only when the tumor was at a distance greater than 1 mm from the resection margin (Konstantinidis *et al.*, 2013). The current evidence shows that only residual tumor of the transection margin (medial resection and pancreatic transection) and not in the mobilization margin (posterior and anterior surface) is associated with a significantly worse prognosis (Jamieson *et al.*, 2010). Analyzing 148 consecutive resections, R1 status (microscopic evidence of tumor < or = 1 mm from the resection margin) was confirmed in 74% of cases. The medial (46%) and the posterior (44%) margins were most commonly involved. The median survival was 18.9 months for R1 mobilization and 11.1 months for R1 transection (p < 0.001). There was no difference in the survival of the R1 mobilization and the R0 group (p = 0.52) (Jamieson *et al.*, 2010).

Recent evidence proved that standardization of histopathological study comes with an increase in the R1 resection rate, from 53% to 85% (Verbeke and Menon, 2009) and from 14% to 76% (Esposito *et al.*, 2008). Maksymov et al. highlights the urgent need for standardized assessment of pancreatoduodenectomy specimens (Maksymov, Hogan and Khalifa, 2013). If they applied the College of the American Pathologists recommendations (assessment only of the bile duct, pancreatic neck and SMA margins) an R1 status would be achieved in 9 out of 25 patients. Extending the examination to the entire retroperitoneal margin (including the SMV margin and the posterior surface of the uncinate process margin) increased the rate of R1 resections to 14 out of 25 cases. Applying the 1–mm rule further increased the number of R1 to 20 of 25 patients (Maksymov, Hogan and Khalifa, 2013).

A French multicenter prospective evaluation of resection margins in 150 specimens of pancreatoduodenectomy found 61% of cases being R1 resections, if the margin was defined as < 1.0 mm (Delpero et al., 2014). The PV-SMV was the most frequently invaded resection margin, in 35% of all patients, and venous resection was the only factor correlated with a higher risk of at least one 0 mm positive resection margin in multivariate analysis (p < 0.001) (Delpero et al., 2014). Two-year progression free survival (PFS) and median PFS time in R0 and R1 (at 0 mm) groups were 42% vs. 26.5%, and 19.5 vs. 10.5 months, respectively (p = 0.02). A positive PV-SMV and SMA margin had significant impact on PFS, whereas a positive posterior margin had no impact (Delpero et al., 2014). However, John et al. found that R1 ≤ 1 mm resection margin does not seem to influence the outcome, while the presence of nodal disease, the number of the lymph nodes involved and the ratio of the number of involved nodes to the number of nodes resected were independent prognostic markers for cancer-specific survival (John et al., 2013).

Jang et al. randomized 200 patients to undergo standard resection or extended resection, with the latter including the dissection of additional lymph nodes and the right half of the nerve plexus around the SMA and celiac axis (Jang et al., 2014). The operation time and the estimated blood loss were higher in the extended resection group. The mean number of lymph nodes retrieved was higher in the extended group (33.7 vs. 17.3, p < 0.001) and the R0 rate was comparable. The median survival after R0 resection was similar between the two groups (18 vs. 19 months, p = 0.239). The conclusion of the authors is that extended lymphadenectomy with dissection of the nerve plexus does not provide a significant survival benefit (Jang et al., 2014).

ARTERY FIRST APPROACH PANCREATICODUODENECTOMY

In a standard pancreatoduodenectomy (sPD) the pancreatic neck is transected, and then the specimen is dissected from the superior mesenteric (SMV) – portal vein (PV) complex, ligating all the small veins draining the pancreatic head. The final step involves separation of the pancreatic head from the superior mesenteric artery (SMA).

Although this can be done multiple ways, the basic principle of an "SMA artery first" approach is early identification of the artery, before the point of no return is reached. The "SMA – first" approach allows an early retropancreatic dissection, especially important when SMA involvement is suspected, reducing the blood loss and resulting in shorter PV clamping times (Rose, 2014).

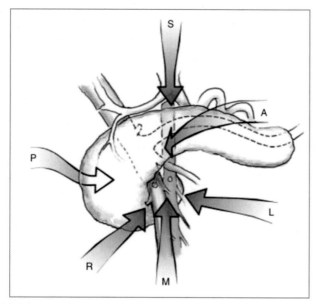

Figure 146. Diagram showing the six approaches to the superior mesenteric artery: S superior approach; A, anterior approach; P, posterior approach; L, left posterior approach; R, right/medial uncinate approach; M, mesenteric approach [Figure reproduced with permission from John Wiley and Sons, from P. Sanjay, K. Takaori, S. Govil, S.V. Shrikhande, J.A. Windsor. "Artery-first" approaches to pancreatoduodenectomy. British Journal of Surgery. 99 (8), 1027–1035, 2012 (Sanjay *et al.*, 2012)].

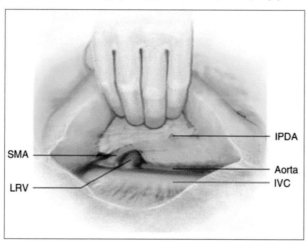

Figure 147. Posterior approach, exposing the origin of superior mesenteric artery (SMA) in front of the left renal vein after kocherization. For clarity the SMA has been made more apparent. IPDA, inferior pancreatoduodenal artery; LRV, left renal vein; IVC, inferior vena cava [Figure reproduced with permission from John Wiley and Sons, from P. Sanjay, K. Takaori, S. Govil, S.V. Shrikhande, J.A. Windsor. "Artery-first" approaches to pancreatoduodenectomy. British Journal of Surgery. 99 (8), 1027–1035, 2012 (Sanjay *et al.*, 2012)].

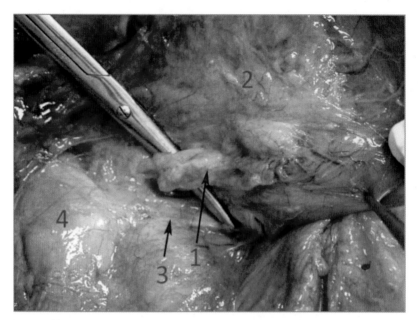

Figure 148. Dissection on a cadaveric model, using a posterior superior mesenteric artery (1) first approach. 2 – posterior surface of the pancreatic head, 3 – left renal vein, 4 – inferior vena cava (Image personal courtesy of SH, IN).

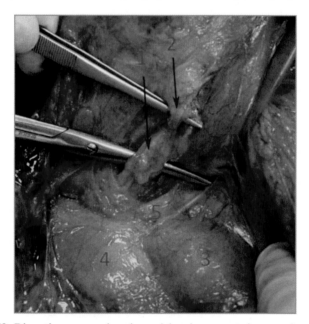

Figure 149. Dissection on a cadaveric model, using a posterior superior mesenteric artery (1) first approach. 2 – inferior pancreaticoduodenl artery, 3 – aorta, 4 – inferior vena cava, 5 – left renal vein (Image personal courtesy of SH, IN).

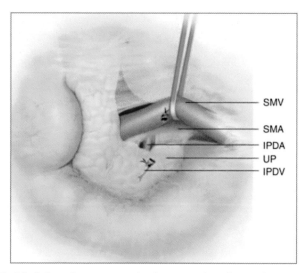

Figure 150. Medial uncinate approach, demonstrating the uncinate process (UP), inferior pancreatoduodenal artery (IPDA) and vein (IPDV), superior mesenteric artery (SMA) and vein (SMV) after kocherization and mobilization of the duodenojejunal flexure [Figure reproduced with permission from John Wiley and Sons, from P. Sanjay, K. Takaori, S. Govil, S.V. Shrikhande, J.A. Windsor. "Artery-first" approaches to pancreatoduodenectomy. British Journal of Surgery. 99 (8), 1027–1035, 2012 (Sanjay *et al.*, 2012)].

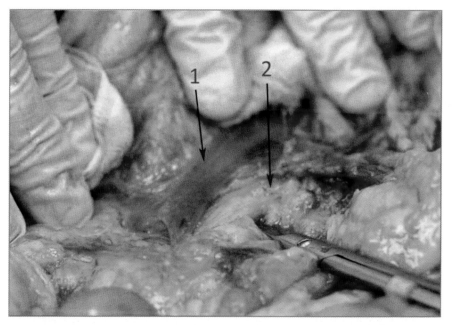

Figure 151. Dissection on a cadaveric model, revealing the superior mesenteric artery (2) by an inferior supracolic approach: 1 – superior mesenteric vein (Image personal courtesy of SH, IN).

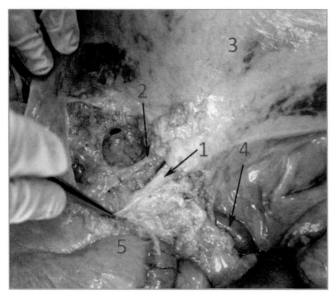

Figure 152. Dissection on a cadaveric model, using a mesenteric superior mesenteric artery first approach: 1 – superior mesenteric artery, 2 – superior mesenteric vein, 3 – transverse mesocolon retracted cephalad, 4 – duodenojejunal angle, 5 – mesentery (Image personal courtesy of SH, IN).

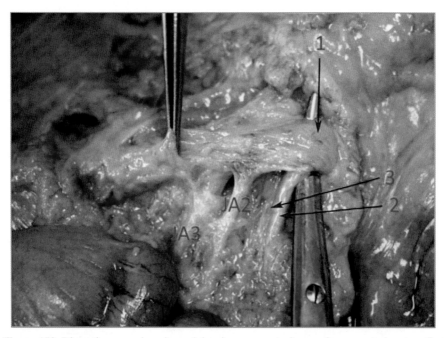

Figure 153. Dissection on cadaveric model, using a mesenteric superior mesenteric artery first approach: 1 – superior mesenteric artery, 2 – first jejunal artery, 3 – first jejunal vein, JA2 and JA3 – second and third jejunal arteries (Image personal courtesy of SH, IN).

SECTION X – THE SPLEEN

*An intimate knowledge of physiology is necessary
to make a successful operator as is anatomy.*

Augustus Charles Bernays

CHAPTER 28

EMBRYOLOGY

RUXANDRA IRINA NEGOI

The spleen starts its embryological development during the fifth week of intrauterine life, from mesenchymal cells located in the dorsal mesogastrium (Moore and Persaud, 2008).

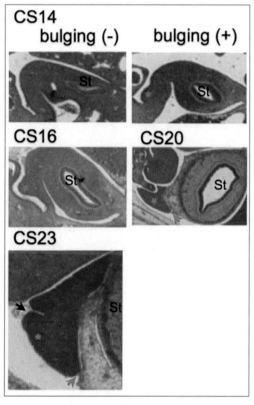

Figure 154. Macroscopic view of the dorsal mesogastrium showing the presence of the spleen or its primordium at Carnegie stages 14, 16, 20, and 23. *, Spleen (primordium); St, stomach; red arrow, segmentation by the folds; black arrow, intrahepatic folds (Figure reproduced with permission from John Wiley and Sons from Aya Endo, Saki Ueno, Shigehito Yamada, Chigako Uwabe, Tetsuya Takakuwa. Morphogenesis of the Spleen During the Human Embryonic Period. The Anatomical Record: Advances in Integrative Anatomy and Evolutionary Biology, 298 (5), 820–826, 2014) (Endo *et al.*, 2015).

The spleen starts its embryological development during the fifth week of intrauterine life, from mesenchymal cells located in the dorsal mesogastrium (Burn et al., 2008). During the "preliminary stage", up to the 14th week, erythrocytes and macrophages are observed into a network of mesenchymal cells. Beginning with the 15th week starts the "transformation stage", with lobules appearance. Theses lobules are centered by a central artery, while at their periphery appears the red pulp. The white pulp appears during the 18th week, during lymphoid colonization of the spleen. During the 23rd week, the primary follicles can be observed (Vellguth, von Gaudecker & Müller-Hermelink, 1985). An evaluation of the morphometric parameters of the spleen showed a length between 3.1 mm and 35.6 mm, correlated with the gestational age of 9 weeks and 40 weeks, respectively (Üngör et al., 2007). Accessory spleens are found in 10–15% of the population, and should be taken into consideration in the differential diagnosis of intra- and peripancreatic tumors (Weiand & Mangold, 2003). In 1–2% of cases can be located inside the pancreatic tail (Weiand & Mangold, 2003).

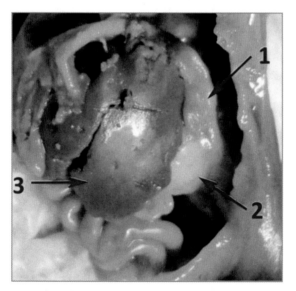

Figure 155. Anatomical dissection of a human embryo demonstrating the spleen (1), the left kidney (2) and the liver (3) (Figure courtesy of RIN).

CHAPTER 29

ANATOMY

IONUȚ NEGOI, MIRCEA BEURAN

The spleen is a solid organ, rich in vascular and lymphatic tissue. Its average size is 12/8/4 cm, with a mean weight in adults of 150 g (Negoi *et al.*, 2010).

EXTERNAL CONFIGURATION

The spleen presents a diaphragmatic and a visceral surface, an upper and a lower margin, and an inferior and a superior pole.

The diaphragmatic surface is convex and smooth, with a superior and lateral orientation. The visceral surface is oriented inferior and medial, and presents centrally the splenic hilum. Around the hilum, the spleen has three concave surfaces, determined by the relationship with the surrounding organs:

- Superiorly with the stomach.
- Inferiorly with the left kidney.
- Anteriorly with the left angle of the colon.

TOPOGRAPHY

The spleen is located in the left upper abdominal quadrant. The anatomical landmarks for its projection on the thoraco-abdominal wall are:

- The ninth rib for the upper splenic margin.
- The eleventh rib for the lower margin.
- The superior pole is located two centimeters lateral to the tenth thoracic vertebra.
- The inferior pole should not overpass the left costal margin.

ANATOMICAL RELATIONSHIPS

The diaphragmatic surface, covered by peritoneum has anatomical relationships with the left pleural recess, the left lung and the ninth to eleventh intercostal spaces. The visceral surface has anatomical relationships with the greater curvature of the stomach, the left kidney and adrenal gland, and the left angle of the colon.

PERITONEUM OF THE SPLEEN

The spleen is covered entirely by visceral peritoneum, closely adherent to its capsule. The reflection of the visceral splenic peritoneum to neighboring organs gives rise to the following peritoneal ligaments:

• The gastrosplenic ligament, located between the splenic hilum and the greater gastric curvature, containing between its layers the short gastric vessels.

• The renolienal ligament, between the splenic hilum and the left kidney, containing the splenic artery, vein and pancreatic tail.

VASCULAR SUPPLY

ARTERIES

The splenic artery is the third branch of the celiac artery, with a diameter greater than the left gastric and common hepatic artery. After its emergence, the splenic artery has a tortuous trajectory along the upper margin of the pancreatic body. It has a length of 10–30 cm, while the mean distance between the aorta and the spleen is 10 cm. From an anatomical point of view three segments may be described:

• The first one, above the pancreas, where is usually located the dorsal pancreatic artery.

• The second one, retropancreatic, located posterior to the body of the pancreas, where may be found the origin of the great pancreatic artery.

• The third segment, anterior to the pancreatic tail, where may be found the origin of the artery of the pancreatic tail (Negoi *et al.*, 2010).

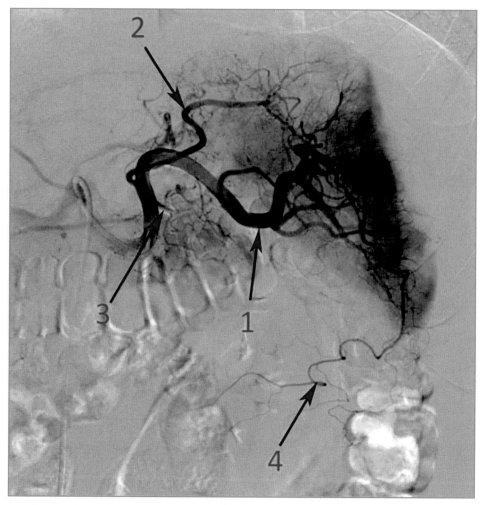

Figure 156. Angiography of the splenic artery (1) revealing the posterior gastric artery (2), dorsal pancreatic artery (3), and left gastroepiploic artery (4) (Figure courtesy of Emergency Hospital of Bucharest, Department of Angiography).

In the splenic hilum, the artery divides into two terminal branches, the superior and the inferior one. Each of these branches will branch off into a polar and a middle branch. According to this vascular distribution, the spleen will present four segments:

- Upper polar.
- Superior and medial.
- Inferior and medial
- Lower polar.

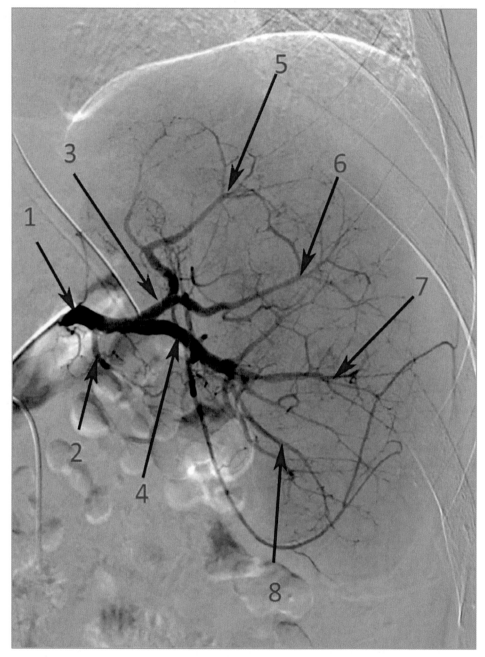

Figure 157. Angiography of the splenic artery (1) revealing the great pancreatic artery (2), the superior (3) and inferior (4) terminal branches, with the four segmental arteries (5 – upper polar, 6 – superior and medial, 7 – inferior and medial, 8 – lower polar) (Figure courtesy of Emergency Hospital of Bucharest, Department of Angiography).

Liu *et al.* studied the vascular anatomy of the spleen in 850 specimens, observing a single lobar artery in 7 cases (0.8%), two lobar arteries in 730 cases (86%), three lobar arteries in 104 cases (12.2%), and multiple lobar arteries (> 3) in 9 cases (1%) (Liu *et al.*, 1996). In a subgroup of 276 cases, the segmental arteries were three in 17%, four in 53%, five in 24%, six in 4%, seven in 1% and eight in 1%. The superior polar artery was found in 31.3%, the inferior polar artery in 38.8%, and both in 13.3% of cases (Liu *et al.*, 1996).

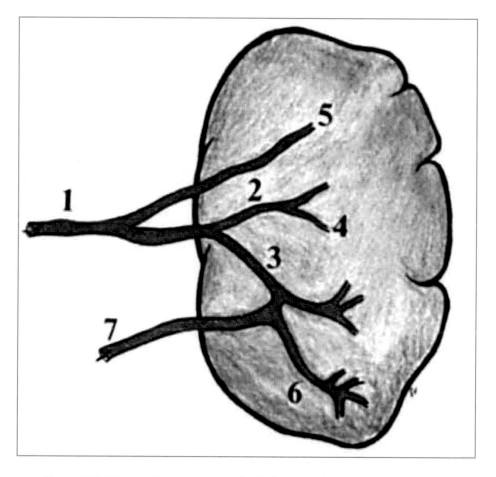

Figure 158. Diagram showing suggested splenic nomenclature: 1, common splenic artery; 2, superior splenic artery; 3, inferior splenic artery; 4, central segmental artery; 5, superior polar artery; 6, inferior polar artery; 7, left gastro-epiploic artery [Figure reproduced with permission from John Wiley and Sons, from H.P. Redmond, J.M. Redmond, B.P. Rooney, J.P. Duignan, D.J. Bouchier-Hayes. Surgical anatomy of the human spleen. British Journal of Surgery, 76, 198–201, 1989 (Redmond *et al.*, 1989)].

Table 14

Origins of the splenic vasculature [Table reproduced with permission from John Wiley and Sons, from H.P. Redmond, J.M. Redmond, B.P. Rooney, J.P. Duignan, D.J. Bouchier-Hayes. Surgical anatomy of the human spleen. British Journal of Surgery, 76, 198–201, 1989 (Redmond *et al.*, 1989)]

Vessel origin	Superior splenic artery	Inferior splenic artery	Superior polar artery	Inferior polar artery	Left gastroepiploic artery
Common splenic artery	100	100	39.8	14.5	35
Superior splenic artery	–	–	60.2	–	6.7
Inferior splenic artery	–	–	–	28	38.3
Superior polar artery	–	–	–	–	–
Inferior polar artery	–	–	–	–	20
Left gastroepiploic artery	–	–	–	57.5	–
The values are percentages					

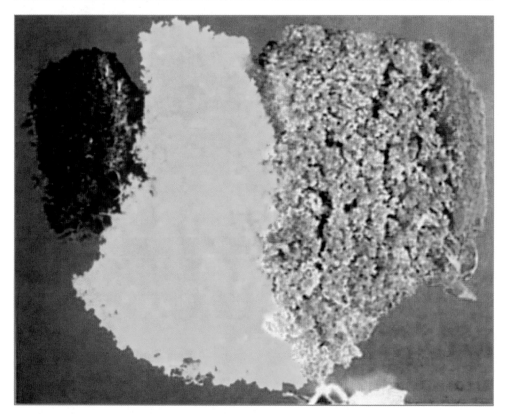

Figure 159. Cast of a spleen containing four segments. Green and red, polar; yellow and blue, central. The avascular planes between segments can be observed [Figure reproduced with permission from John Wiley and Sons, from H.P. Redmond, J.M. Redmond, B.P. Rooney, J.P. Duignan, D.J. Bouchier-Hayes. Surgical anatomy of the human spleen. British Journal of Surgery, 76, 198–201, 1989 (Redmond *et al.*, 1989)].

VEINS

In the splenic hilum, two-three venous branches give rise to the splenic vein. This has a straight trajectory on the posterior surface of the pancreatic body. Posterior to the pancreatic neck it joins the superior mesenteric vein to give rise to the portal vein.

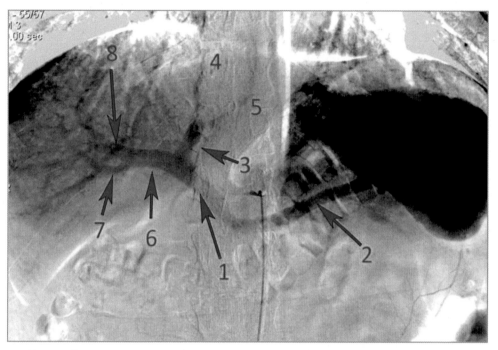

Figure 160. Portography (1) revealing the splenic vein (2), left portal vein (3), left portal vein segmental branches for segments 2 (4) and 3 (5), right branch of the portal vein (6) with right posterior (7) and right anterior sectional branches (8) (Figure courtesy of Emergency Hospital of Bucharest, Department of Angiography).

INNERVATION

The spleen receives sympathetic and parasympathetic fibers from the celiac plexus.

CHAPTER 30

HISTOLOGY

SORIN HOSTIUC, VALENTIN ENACHE

The spleen has two main parts that are visible macroscopically – the white pulp and the red pulp.

The white pulp contains mainly the following structures:

• B-cell follicle – a round area of small lymphocytes that is surrounded by medium lymphocytes; it is the area responsible for the production of memory cells and immunoglobulin producing cells.

• T-cell area – an irregular area of small lymphocytes, mostly CD4+.

• The perifollicular area – it separates the red from the white pulp and contains a high number of red blood cells.

The red pulp contains the following structures:

• Sinuses – a network of sinuses with an interrupted basement membrane and leaky capillaries, which allows the passage of red blood cells between the sinuses and the cords.

• Splenic cords (Billroth's cords) – contain macrophages that filter red blood cells and ingest the senescent or damaged ones.

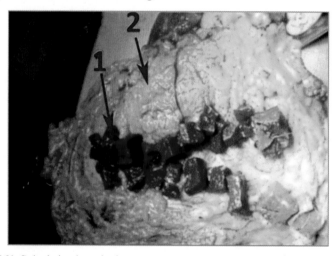

Figure 161. Splenic implants in the greater omentum – arrangement in two parallel lines (Figure reproduced with permission from Al.L. Chiotoroiu, D.M. Venter, I. Negoi, C. Vârtosu, O. Plotogea, S. Păun, M. Vartic, M. Beuran. Splenic Implant Assessment in Trauma, Chirurgia, 109 (6), 731–740, 2014) (Chiotoroiu *et al.*, 2014).

In trauma patients with splenic injuries, who can not be managed by a selective nonoperative management (Beuran *et al.*, 2010) or by a spleen-preserving surgical technique, splenic fragments can be implanted into the greater omentum. This surgical technique seems to partially restore the immunological functions of the spleen, correlating with the effort to prevent overwhelming postsplenectomy sepsis (OPSI) (Chiotoroiu *et al.*, 2014).

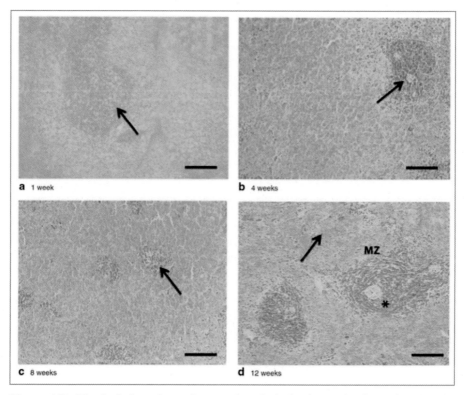

Figure 162. Histological sections of autogenic splenic implants, showing a lymphocytic aggregate of follicular aspect (arrow) at 1 week; b lymphocytic infiltrate (arrow) at 4 weeks; c lymphoid follicle with central arteriole (arrow), and the outline of red and white pulp at 8 weeks; and d well defined red and white pulp (arrow and asterisk respectively) and a marginal zone (MZ) at 12 weeks (haematoxylin and eosin stain, scale bar 50 μm) (Figure reproduced with permission from John Wiley and Sons, from R.G. Marques, S.B.S.G. Lucena, C.E.R. Caetano, V. Oliveira de Sousa, M.C. Portela, A. Petroianu. Blood clearance of Howell–Jolly bodies in an experimental autogenic splenic implant model. British Journal of Surgery. Apr. 23, 2014) (Marques *et al.*, 2014).

SECTION XI – THE SMALL BOWEL

Everything has been written but not everything has been read.

Bernard Cristalli

CHAPTER 31

EMBRYOLOGY

RUXANDRA IRINA NEGOI

The upper anatomical boundary of the midgut is represented by the midpoint of the duodenal loop and the inferior one by the primitive colic flexure, which later becomes the left colic flexure (Negoi *et al.*, 2010). The midgut derivatives are the small bowel (inferior to the ampulla of Vater) and the right colon (cecum, vermiform appendix, ascending colon and right two thirds of the transverse colon). All of these structures will be vascularized by the superior mesenteric artery.

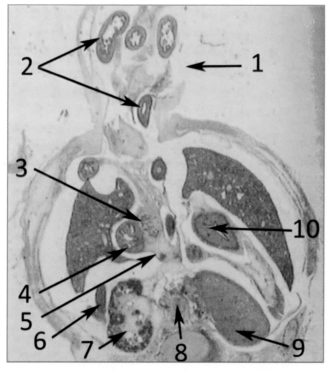

Figure 163. Transverse section through the abdomen of a rat embryo revealing the physiologic umbilical herniation (1), herniated bowel loops, pancreatic head (3), duodenum (4), mesopancreatoduodenum (5), gonads (6), kidney (7), aorta (8) and kidney (9) (Figure personal courtesy of RIN).

During its embryological development, the midgut increases rapidly in length, giving rise to the primary intestinal loop. From the upper arm of the primary intestinal loop develops the lower part of the duodenum, jejunum and the upper ileum. The lower arm will develop into the last 80 cm of ileum and the right colon. The top of the loop is connected with the yolk sac through the vitelline duct. The vitelline duct will obliterate during intrauterine life. In cases of failure of the vitelline duct to obliterate there will appear Meckel's diverticulum, 40–80 cm from the ileocecal valve.

The small bowel loops, liver and mesonephros will grow faster than the abdominal cavity. Thus, during the sixth week of intrauterine life physiologic umbilical herniation occurs. During this process the intestinal loops herniate outside the abdominal cavity, through the umbilical ring, into the amniotic cavity.

Starting with the tenth intrauterine week, the bowel loops increase in number, and the cecum diverticulum appears at the lower arm of the intestinal loop. Concomitantly with this process of physiologic herniation, the primary intestinal loop rotates in the axis of the superior mesenteric artery, 270 counterclockwise from a frontal view.

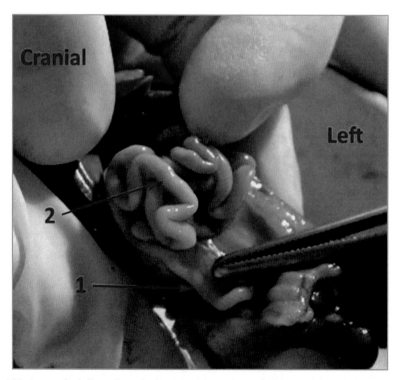

Figure 164. Anatomical dissection of a human embryo demonstrating a right sided descending and sigmoid colon (1); 2 - small bowel loops (Figure courtesy of RIN).

During the tenth week, with involution of the mesonephros and further development of the abdominal cavity, the herniated intestine returns to the abdominal cavity, in a very precise order (Moore and Persaud, 2008):

Firstly, will return the future jejunal loops, passing posteriorly to the superior mesenteric artery (Moore and Persaud, 2008). They will occupy the left side of the abdomen, compressing on the posterior abdominal wall, the hindgut, which will later become the descending colon.

Secondly, the future ileal loops will return, which will occupy the right side of the abdominal cavity.

The last returned segment is the lower arm of the intestinal loop, which will occupy a transverse position, with the cecal diverticulum in the subhepatic space. This segment will give rise to the two right thirds of the transverse colon. The cecal diverticulum undergoes a descension into the right iliac fossa, giving rise to the hepatic flexure of the colon, ascending colon and cecum. The apex of the cecal diverticulum does not increase in dimension, forming the vermiform appendix.

During the cecal descension, the vermiform appendix increases in length. While the cecum is descending, the vermiform appendix may take a posterior position (retrocecal or retrocolic). At birth the vermiform appendix is a tubular structure, extending inferiorly from the cecum. Through unequal growth of the cecum walls, the origin of the vermiform appendix will become located on the medial wall of the cecum. By compression of the small bowel loops, the ascending colon will become a secondary retroperitoneal organ. Its coalescence fascia is termed Toldt I, while the coalescence fascia of the descending colon is termed Toldt II.

CHAPTER 32
ANATOMY

IONUȚ NEGOI, MIRCEA BEURAN, SORIN PĂUN

BOUNDARIES

The superior limit of the small bowel is the duodenojejunal angle of Treitz, projected onto the posterior abdominal wall on the left of the second lumbar vertebra. Inferiorly, the limit is represented by the ilocecal valve, located in the right iliac fossa. The small bowel is an intraperitoneal organ with a length of 300–800 cm. Its diameter decreases from 2.5–3 cm in the jejunum, to 1.5–2 cm in the ileum (Negoi et al., 2010). Current evidence suggests that as much as 50% of the small bowel can be resected, without impairment of its function. There is no clear boundary between the two small bowel segments, the jejunum usually being the superior three fifths.

TOPOGRAPHY AND ANATOMICAL RELATIONSHIPS

The jejunum and ileum are intraperitoneal organs, located in the inframesocolic space. They project onto the anterior abdominal wall in the periumbilical, left and right lower quadrants.

The anatomical relationships of the small bowel are:

Anteriorly: the greater omentum and anterior abdominal wall.

Posteriorly, the jejunum has anatomical relationships with the lower pole of the left kidney, the left ureter, the left genital vessels and the inferior mesenteric vein. On the midline, the small bowel has relationships with the aorta, the inferior vena cava, the left lumbar sympathetic chain, the third duodenal segment and the pancreatic head. The ileum has posterior relationships with the lower pole of the right kidney, the right ureter and the right genital vessels.

Superiorly located is the transverse colon with its mesocolon.

Inferiorly, it has anatomical relationships with the cecum, the vermiform appendix and the sigmoid colon. Below the superior pelvic brim, the inferior ileum has relationships with the urinary bladder, the posterior surface of the uterus and the rectum (Negoi et al., 2010).

MESENTERY

The small bowel mesentery may be described as having two margins (a posterior or its root and an anterior or its intestinal side) and two surfaces (a right and a left one). While the intestinal margin has a length corresponding to the small bowel, its root is 18–20 cm long. Three segments of the mesentery root can be described:

- A first oblique one, from the right of the duodenojejunal angle to the upper margin of the third duodenal segment.
- A second vertical one, which crosses the anterior surface of the third duodenal segment. At this level, the superior mesenteric vessels join the mesentery.
- The third oblique segment, from the inferior margin of the third duodenal segment to the ileocolic angle. This segment intersects the retroperitoneal structures, such as the inferior vena cava, the right ureter and the right genital vessels (Negoi et al., 2010).

VASCULAR SUPPLY

ARTERIES

The small bowel receives its vascular supply from the superior mesenteric artery. The superior mesenteric artery is the second major visceral branch of the abdominal aorta, having its origin 1–2 cm inferior to the celiac artery. According to its trajectory, the superior mesenteric artery presents three segments:

- The retropancreatic segment, located posterior to the pancreatic neck. This arterial segment is surrounded by the following venous structures: (a) on the right – the superior mesenteric vein, (b) on the left – the inferior mesenteric vein, (c) superiorly – the splenic vein, (d) inferiorly – the left renal vein.
- The preduodenal segment, anterior to the third duodenal segment and the uncinate process of the pancreas. This arterial segment has anatomical relationships anterior and to the right with the superior mesenteric vein.
- The intra-mesentery segment, located in the root of the mesentery.

The superior mesenteric artery left branches supply the small bowel, while the right branches the right colon. Its right sided branches are:

- Inferior pancreaticoduodenal artery.
- Middle colic artery.
- Right colic artery.
- Ileocolic artery.

The small bowel branches are variable as numbers, 8–17. After a trajectory into the small bowel mesentery they divide into ascending and descending branches. These branches make arterial arcades:

- The first four arterial branches give rise to one arterial arcade.
- The 4th–8th branches give rise to two arterial arcades.
- The remaining branches form two or three arterial arcades.

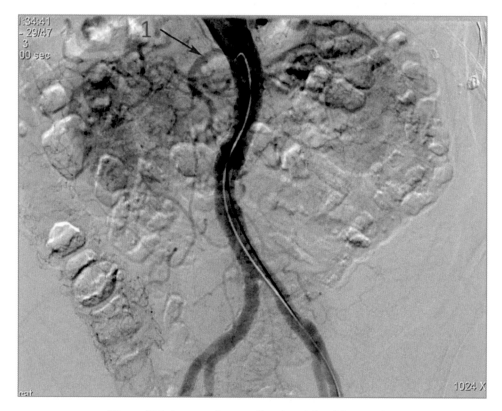

Figure 165. Aortography revealing the origin of the superior mesenteric artery (1) (Figure courtesy of Emergency Hospital of Bucharest, Department of Angiography).

The last ileal segment presents a poorer blood supply, through a single arterial arcade. This vascular arcade is formed by the anastomosis between the last ileal artery and the recurrent branch of the ileocolic artery. The closest vascular arcade from the intestinal wall is termed the marginal arcade. The marginal arcade is 4–5 cm from the jejunum and 1–2 cm from the ileal wall. The marginal arcade branches off the terminal straight arteries (Negoi *et al.*, 2010).

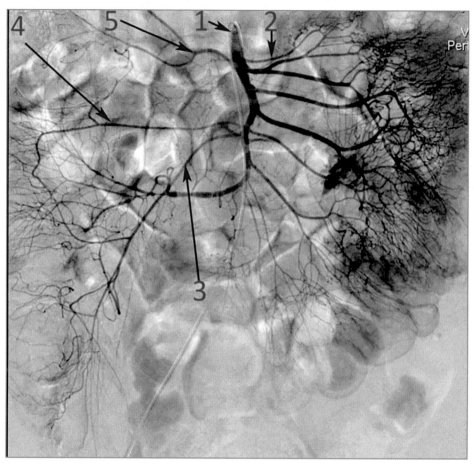

Figure 166. Angiography of the superior mesenteric artery (1) revealing the first jejunal artery (2), ileocolic artery (3), right colic artery (4) and middle colic artery (5) (Figure courtesy of Emergency Hospital of Bucharest, Department of Angiography).

VEINS

Venous drainage of the jejunum and ileum is homonymous to the arterial supply. The superior mesenteric vein is formed by two roots, a right and a left. The right root receives the ileocolic, the right colic, the middle colic and the gastrocolic trunk of Henle. The gastrocolic trunk is formed by the right gastro-epiploic, the superior anterior pancreaticoduodenal and the right superior colic veins.

The left root of the inferior mesenteric vein is formed by the ileal and jejunal branches.

LYMPHATICS

The small bowel has a very rich network of lymphatics, with their origin in the intestinal villi.

INNERVATION

The small intestine receives its vegetative innervation from the superior mesenteric plexus. The nerve fibers reach the jejunum and ileum through peri-arterial nerve plexuses, which accompany the superior mesenteric artery branches (Negoi *et al.*, 2010).

CHAPTER 33

HISTOLOGY

SORIN HOSTIUC, MONICA POPIEL

The small bowel contains mainly four basic layers: mucosa, submucosa, muscularis and adventitia.

The mucosa has a series of adaptations aimed toward increasing the surface area, needed for the transfer of nutrients. The mucosa contains three sub-layers: epithelium, lamina propria and muscularis mucosa. The epithelium and the lamina propria form luminal projections called villi. The epithelium, containing unicellular, cylindrical epithelial cells, is divided into two sub-compartments: villous and cryptic.

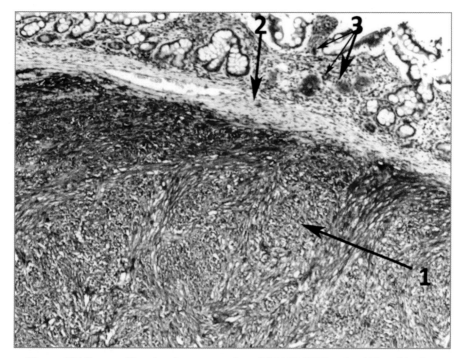

Figure 167. Immunohistochemistry expression of CD117 (KIT), using 100 × objective. Small bowel GIST tumor cells (1) and normal mucosal mast cells (3) showing immunoreactivity, while the muscularis mucosa shows the absence of reactivity (2) (Image courtesy of VE, used with permission).

The villous compartment contains tall, cylindrical cells, with a brush-like apical surface formed by structures known as microvilli. The crypt epithelium has mainly a regenerative function for the villous epithelium. Particular to the lamina propria is a high number of immune cells (plasma cells, mast cells, eosinophils, histiocytes, and lymphocytes. The muscularis mucosa is a thin layer containing elastic fibers and smooth muscle fibers.

The submucosa is a paucicellular layer built around a network of collagen and elastic fibers. At this level, a large number of vessels and Meissner's plexus, one of the two main myenteric plexi (together with Auerbach's plexus from the muscle layer) are identifiable.

The muscular layer is represented by a thicker, outer layer of smooth muscle cells, containing two sublayers: one longitudinal (external) and one circular (internal), between which the myenteric plexus of Auerbach and Interstitial Cajal cells are identifiable.

The serosa covers the external surface of the small bowel and contains a layer of flat-cuboidal mesothelial cells, under which a layer of loose connective tissue (subserosal layer) is found.

SECTION XII – THE APPENDIX

The appendix is generally attached to the cecum.

Mark Ravitch

CHAPTER 34
EMBRYOLOGY

RUXANDRA IRINA NEGOI

The cecum, the vermiform appendix, the ascending colon and the two right thirds of the transverse colon have their embryological origin in the midgut. Their embryological development was presented in the small bowel chapter (Negoi *et al.*, 2010).

CHAPTER 35

ANATOMY

IONUȚ NEGOI, MIRCEA BEURAN, REGINA KIRBY

The vermiform appendix, with a length of 2–20 cm, has its opening on the posterior-medial wall of the cecum, around 2 cm lower than the ileocecal valve (Negoi *et al.*, 2010). It is an intraperitoneal organ, presenting its own mesentery, termed the mesoappendix.

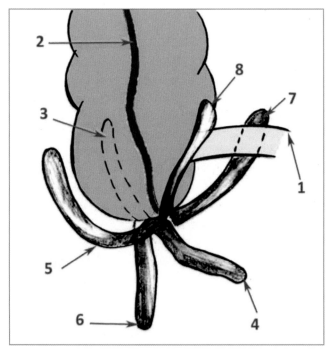

Figure 168. Schematic representation of different possibilities of disposition for the vermiform appendix: 1 – last ileal loop, 2 – anterior colon tenia, 3 – retrocecal, 4 – mediocecal, 5 – laterocecal, 6 – infracecal, 7 – retroileal, 8 – preileal [Image personal courtesy of IN, used with permission from (Negoi *et al.*, 2010)].

The vermiform appendix has in up to 75% of cases a retrocecal or retrocolic position, but may be found in pelvic (around 20%) retro- or preileal (5%) positions.

PROJECTION ON THE ANTERIOR
ABDOMINAL WALL

The vermiform appendix is projected into the right iliac fossa, where has been described the following painful points during acute appendicitis:
- McBurney's point is located on the spino-umbilical line, at the meeting point between the lateral one third with the medial two thirds.

ANATOMICAL RELATIONSHIPS

Anteriorly: the ileum loops and the anterior abdominal wall.
Laterally: the cecum.
Posteriorly: the iliopsoas muscle, the femoral nerve, and the external iliac vessels.

VASCULAR SUPPLY

ARTERIES

The vermiform appendix receives its arterial supply via the appendicular artery, a branch of the ileocolic artery. The ileocolic artery, branching off from the superior mesenteric artery, has a trajectory inferiorly and to the right. It divides into the following branches:
- The recurrent ileal artery, which anastomoses with the last ileal artery, giving rise to the last vascular arcade for the ileum.
- The ascending colic artery, which anastomoses with the descending branch of the right colic artery.
- The anterior cecal artery.
- The posterior cecal artery.
- The appendicular artery, with a trajectory posterior to the ileum, then into the mesoapendix (Negoi et al., 2010).

VEINS

The venous drainage of the vermiform appendix is to veins homonymous to the corresponding arteries.

LYMPHATICS

The lymphatic drainage is to the anterior and posterior cecal lymph nodes, then to the ileocolic and the superior mesenteric lymph nodes.

INNERVATION

Innervation is both sympathetic and parasympathetic, the origin of the fibers being in the superior mesenteric plexus.

CHAPTER 36
HISTOLOGY

VALENTIN ENACHE, IOAN T NASE

The vermiform appendix has a microscopic appearance similar to the colon, with abundant lymphatic tissue in the submucosal layer.

The appendix (vermiform appendix) was for a long time considered as a vestigial structure; however, due to the presence of rich and highly organized lymphoid tissue it is now considered to be involved in mucosal immunity. Similar to all other lower gastrointestinal structures, it consists of four main layers:

Mucosa, with a unilayer of cylindrical cells, sits on a lamina propria, that is rich in lymphoid cells which often distorts the luminal circumference. Underneath the muscularis mucosa is identifiable, a thin band of fibro-muscular tissue, that is discontinuous in the area of the lymphoid follicles, unlike the rest of the colon in which it is continuous.

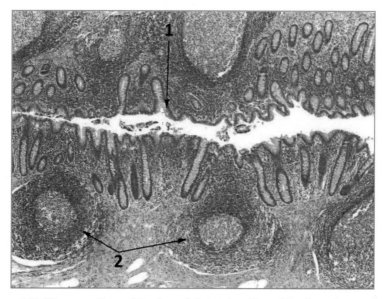

Figure 169. Hematoxylin and Eosin staining using 50 × objective of normal cecal appendix: 1 – normal appendicular mucosa, 2 – lymphoid follicles
(Image courtesy of VE, used with permission).

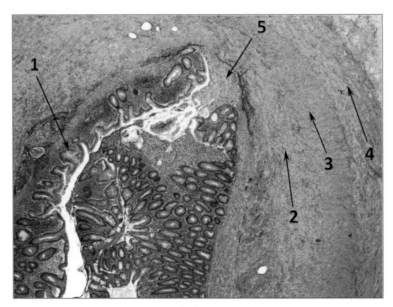

Figure 170. Hematoxylin and Eosin staining using 2.5 × objective of acute appendicitis: 1 – appendicular mucosa, 2 – submucosa, 3 – circular muscular layer, 4 – longitudinal muscular layer, 5 – infiltration of neutrophils into the mucosa, defining acute inflammation (Image courtesy of VE, used with permission).

Submucosa – is a loose conjunctive tissue containing numerous collagen and elastic fibers and fibrous cells. Also identifiable are vessels, Meissner's plexus, and nerve fibers.

Muscle layer – is thick, consisting of longitudinal and circular fibers separated by a thin layer in which Auerbach's plexus is identifiable.

The serous layer contains a single layer of cuboid, mesothelial cells, covered by a band of fibrous tissue.

SECTION XIII – THE COLON

In anatomy is better to have learned and lost,
than never to have learned at all.

W. Somerset Maugham

CHAPTER 37

EMBRYOLOGY

RUXANDRA IRINA NEGOI

The hindgut has its superior boundary at the primary colic flexure, and inferiorly at the cloaca (Negoi et al., 2010). The hindgut derivatives are the left third of the transverse colon, the descending colon, the sigmoid colon, and the rectum above the dentate line. The artery that supplies all of the embryological derivatives of the hindgut is the inferior mesenteric artery. The hindgut ends in the cloaca, an endodermal region closed inferiorly by the cloacal membrane. In the anterior part of the cloaca is the opening of allantois, the primordium of the urinary bladder. Between the hindgut and the allantois will develop the urorectal septum. Secondary to this process, the cloaca will be divided into an anterior space, the urogenital sinus and a posterior space, the anorectal sinus.

The anorectal sinus gives rise to the rectum and the anal canal above the dentate line. These anatomical structures, embryologically derived from endoderm, presents a single layer of cylindrical epithelium in their mucosa. They are also vascularized by the inferior mesenteric vessels, the lymphatic drainage is accomplished by the inferior mesenteric lymph nodes, and the innervation is via the inferior hypogastric plexus (Sadler, 2009).

The anal canal, below the dentate line, has as its embryological origin the proctodeum, an ectodermal structure. According to this, it will have a mucosa with stratified squamous epithelium, will be vascularized by the inferior rectal arteries, the lymphatic drainage will be accomplished by the superficial inguinal lymph nodes, and will have somatic innervation. The boundary between these two areas is the dentate or pectinate line. These differences in blood supply and lymphatic drainage are clinically important when considering dissemination pathways for rectal cancers.

CHAPTER 38

ANATOMY

IONUȚ NEGOI, MIRCEA BEURAN

The large intestine extends from the ileocecal valve to the anus, having an average length of 1.5 m. The large bowel is topographically divided into the cecum, the ascending, transverse, descending and sigmoid colon, and the rectum.

CECUM

The cecum is the first segment of the large bowel, around 6–7 cm in length (Negoi *et al.*, 2010). Although usually located in the right iliac fossa, its position varies widely, from the subhepatic to the pelvic space.

ANATOMICAL RELATIONSHIPS

Anteriorly: the anterior abdominal wall.
Posteriorly: the iliopsoas muscle, the femoral nerve, and the lateral femoral cutaneous nerve.
Laterally: the iliac muscle, and the lateral half of the inguinal area.
Medially: the last ileal loop, the vermiform appendix, the external iliac vessels, the right ureter and the right genital vessels.

ASCENDING COLON

The ascending colon is a secondary retroperitoneal organ, and has a mean length of 10–15 cm.

ANATOMICAL RELATIONSHIPS

Anteriorly: the anterior abdominal wall.
Posteriorly: the quadratus lumborum muscle, the subcostal, iliohypogastric and ilioinguinal nerves, and the right kidney.

Laterally: the lateral abdominal wall, delimitating the right paracolic gutter.

Medially: the small bowel, the duodenum, the inferior vena cava, the right ureter and the right genital vessels.

TRANSVERSE COLON

The transverse colon extends between the right and left colic flexures, it has a mean length of 50 cm, and is an intraperitoneal organ.

ANATOMICAL RELATIONSHIPS

Anteriorly: the anterior abdominal wall.

Posteriorly: the right kidney, the duodenum, the pancreatic head and body, the left kidney.

Superiorly: the visceral surface of the right hemiliver, the gastric antrum, the lower pole of the spleen.

Inferiorly: the small bowel loops.

DESCENDING COLON

The descending colon, with a mean length of 10–25 cm, is a secondary retroperitoneal organ attached to the posterior abdominal wall through the Toldt II coalescence fascia.

ANATOMICAL RELATIONSHIPS

Anteriorly: the abdominal wall.

Posteriorly: the quadratus lumborum muscle, the subcostal, iliohypogastric and ilioinguinal nerves.

Laterally: the lateral abdominal wall, delimitating the left paracolic gutter.

Medially: the jejunal loops, the fourth duodenal segment, the inferior mesenteric vein, the aorta, the left ureteral and the left genital vessels.

SIGMOID COLON

The sigmoid colon is an intraperitoneal organ, extending from the iliac crest to the third sacral vertebra. It has a mean length of 50 cm (Negoi *et al.*, 2010).

ANATOMICAL RELATIONSHIPS

Anteriorly: the anterior abdominal wall, and the ileal loops.

Posteriorly: the iliopsoas muscle, the common and external iliac vessels, the femoral and genitofemoral nerves, the left ureter and the left genital vessels.

Laterally: the iliac muscle, the lateral half of the inguinal area, the external iliac vessels and the obturator nerve.

Medially: the ileal loops.

Inferiorly: the urinary bladder and the uterus.

SIGMOID MESOCOLON

Its root has an inverted *V* shape, with two branches:

• An initial ascending one, parallel to the left external and common iliac arteries.

• A descending one, which intersects the common iliac artery and vein, and ends at the level of the third sacral vertebra.

Between these two branches the left ureter is located.

VASCULAR SUPPLY OF THE COLON

ARTERIES

The right colon (cecum, ascending colon and right two thirds of the transverse) is vascularized by the superior mesenteric artery, while the left colon (left third of the transverse, descending and sigmoid colon) by the inferior mesenteric artery (Negoi *et al.*, 2010).

SUPERIOR MESENTERIC ARTERY

The colic branches of the superior mesenteric artery are:

• The ileocolic artery, which divides into anterior and posterior cecal arteries and the ascending colic artery.

• The right colic artery, which divides into an ascending and a descending branch.

• The middle colic artery, which emerges immediately below the pancreatic neck. Inside the transverse mesocolon it divides into a right and left branch.

INFERIOR MESENTERIC ARTERY

The inferior mesenteric artery branches off of the aorta, 3–4 cm above its bifurcation, below the third duodenal segment, at the level of the third lumbar vertebra.

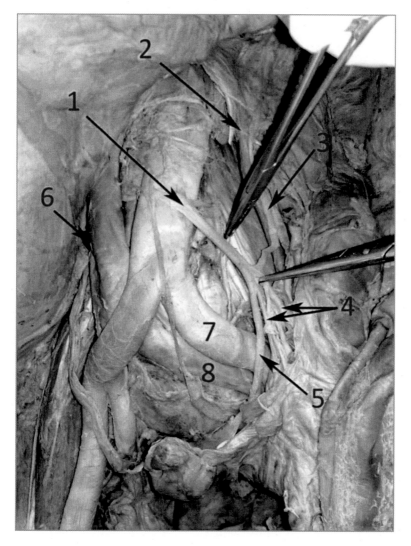

Figure 171. Dissection on a cadaveric model of the inferior mesenteric artery (1) and inferior mesenteric vein (2). 3 – left colic artery, 4 – sigmoidian arteries, 5 – superior rectal artery, 6 – inferior vena cava, 7 – left common iliac artery, 8 – left common iliac vein (Image courtesy of IN).

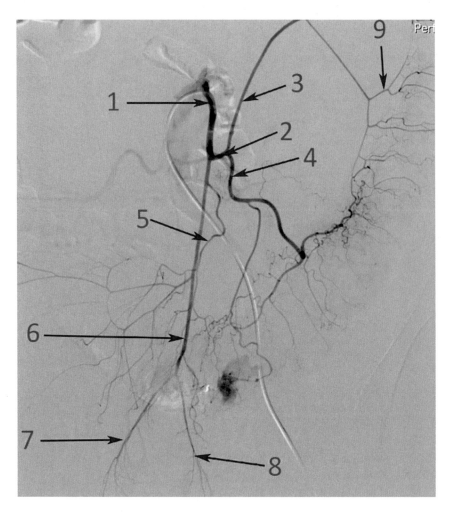

Figure 172. Angiography of the inferior mesenteric artery (1) revealing the left colic artery (2) with its ascending (3) and descending (4) branches, sigmoidian arteries (5), superior rectal artery (6) with its right (7) and left (8) branches. 9 – straight colic arteries. (Figure courtesy of Emergency Hospital of Bucharest, Department of Angiography).

Its branches are the:

• Left colic artery, which emerges 1–2 cm from the inferior mesenteric artery origin. It divides into an ascending and descending branch. The ascending branch has a parallel trajectory with the inferior mesenteric vein.

• Sigmoidian arteries, with a variable numbers of one – nine. They divide into ascending and descending branches.

• Superior rectal artery.

The branches of bifurcation of the ileocolic, right colic, middle colic, left colic and sigmoidian arteries are anastomosing, giving rise to the vascular arcade of Drummond. This is located 1–8 cm from the colonic wall. From the vascular arcade of Drummond emerges the straight colic arteries, which penetrate the colon wall.

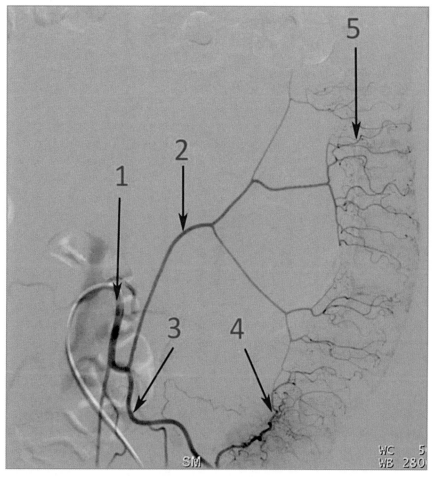

Figure 173. Angiography of the inferior mesenteric artery (1) revealing the left colic artery with its ascending (2) and descending (3) branches, marginal arcade of Drummond (4) and straight colic arteries (5) (Figure courtesy of Emergency Hospital of Bucharest, Department of Angiography).

VEINS

Venous drainage is homonymous to the corresponding arteries, and drains into the superior or inferior mesenteric veins.

The inferior mesenteric vein continues the trajectory of the superior rectal vein. It receives the sigmoidian and the left colic veins. After a parallel course with the fourth duodenal segment it has a retropancreatic trajectory, draining into the splenic, superior mesenteric or portal vein.

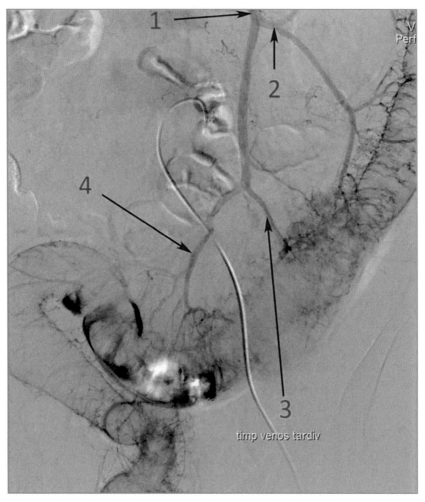

Figure 174. Angiography of the inferior mesenteric artery with late image acquisition, revealing the inferior mesenteric vein (1), the left colic vein (2), sigmoidian vein (3) and upper rectal vein (4) (Figure courtesy of Emergency Hospital of Bucharest, Department of Angiography).

LYMPHATICS

The regional lymph nodes of the colon that drain lymph from the colon are divided into four groups:

- Epicolics – below the colon serosa.
- Paracolics – along the marginal artery of Drummond.
- Intermediates – along the branches of the superior mesenteric artery.
- Central – at the origin of the mesenteric arteries.

The complete mesocolic excision (CME) with central vascular ligation (CVL) represents an extension to colonic cancer resection of the already standardized resection for rectal cancer, having the same guiding principle that surgical sharp dissection, following embryological planes, should improve the oncological outcomes (Negoi *et al.*, 2015a).

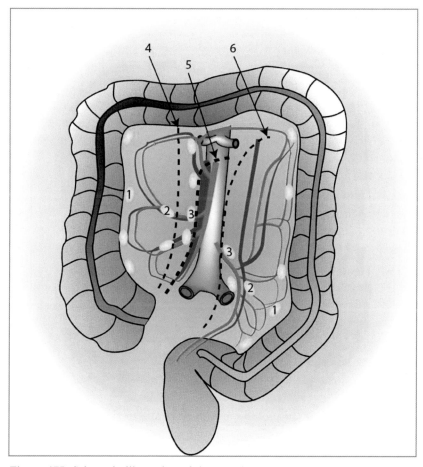

Figure 175. Schematic illustration of the complete mesocolic excision with central vascular ligation for right sided colonic cancer (5) or left colonic tumors (6). According to the Japanese Society for Cancer of the Colon and Rectum (JSCCR) the lymph nodes are classified in D1 (pericolic) – 1; D2 (intermediate) – 2; and D3 (central nodes) – 3. It may observed the equivalence between the Western CME with CVL and the Eastern D3 lymphadenectomy [Personal drawing IN, (Negoi *et al.*, 2015a)].

In 2007, Hohenberger *et al.* from Erlangen, Germany published the technical details of a new concept, termed complete mesocolic excision and central ligation for colonic cancer (Hohenberger, Merkel and Weber, 2007). During CME with CVL for right sided tumors the following should be ligated at their origin from the superior mesenteric artery, the ileocolic and if present, the right colic artery (Negoi *et al.*, 2015a).

Transverse colon tumors require transection of the middle colic artery at its origin. For left sided tumors the inferior mesenteric artery should be transected at its origin from the aorta (West *et al.*, 2012). Using CME and CVL, the group from Erlangen, reported a reduction in the local 5-year recurrence rate from 6.5% to 3.6% and an increase in cancer related, 5-year survival rate from 82.1% to 89.1% (Hohenberger *et al.*, 2009). This specimen oriented technique is associated with removal of more tissue compared to standard surgery, a wider distance from the tumor to the higher vascular tie (131 *vs.* 90 mm, $p < 0.0001$), a longer length of large bowel (314 *vs.* 206 mm, $p < 0.0001$), a wider area of removed mesentery (19657 *vs.* 11829 mm^2, $p < 0.0001$) and a greater lymph node yield (30 *versus* 18, $p < 0.0001$) (West *et al.*, 2010a). These may partially explain the higher reported survival rates with CME and CVL (Negoi *et al.*, 2015a).

It should be noticed the similarities between D3 lymphadenectomy, recommended as standard of care for stage II and III colon cancer in Eastern countries, and Western CME (West *et al.*, 2012; Watanabe *et al.*, 2012). The Japanese nomenclature includes D1 as pericolic (close to the bowel wall), D2 as intermediate (along the feeding artery) and D3 as main (at the origin of the feeding artery) lymph nodes. For right sided tumors D3 lymphadenectomy requires the transection of the feeding arteries next to their origin from the superior mesenteric artery. In left sided cancers a D3 lymphadenectomy requires transection of the IMA close to its aortic origin (Higuchi and Sugihara, 2010).

INNERVATION

The colon receives parasympathetic and sympathetic autonomic innervation.

RIGHT COLON

Sympathetic innervation comes from the superior mesenteric plexus. This plexus receives its fibers from the splanchnic nerves, through the celiac plexus. Parasympathetic fibers originate in the vagal trunks, through the superior mesenteric plexus.

LEFT COLON

Sympathetic innervation comes from the lumbar splanchnic nerves into the preaortic plexus. From this plexus, through the periarterial inferior mesenteric plexus, the fibers reach the left colon. Parasympathetic fibers come through the pelvic splanchnic nerves from the S2 – S4 spinal cord. At this level they pass through the inferior hypogastric plexus, then to the hypogastric nerves, the superior hypogastric plexus, and then via the periarterial plexuses they reach the left colon.

CHAPTER 39
HISTOLOGY

VALENTIN ENACHE, SORIN HOSTIUC

Even if it has a series of regional particularities, most elements are identifiable in all colonic structures, including the rectum, and will be presented together.

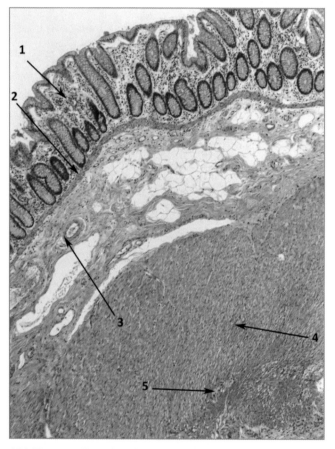

Figure 176. Hematoxylin and Eosin staining using 50x objective of normal colon: 1 – colon mucosa, 2 – muscularis mucosa, 3 – submucosa, 4 – inner circular muscular layer, 5 – myenteric nervous plexus of Auerbach (Image courtesy of VE, used with permission).

The mucosal layer contains at the surface a unilayer of cylindrical cells, covered typically by a very rich glycocalyx that is involved in aiding the commensal bacteria to form a barrier. These cells form crypts that have a unilayer of epithelial cells situated on a basement membrane, and a variable cellular and vascular lamina propria. Epithelial cells are of various types including absorptive colonocytes, goblet cells, endocrine cells, Paneth's cells, M cells, follicle associated epithelium, or inflammatory cells.

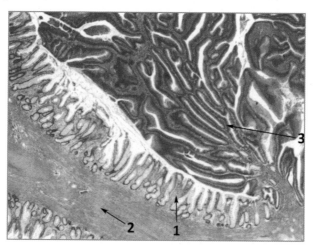

Figure 177. Hematoxylin and Eosin staining using 50 × objective of colonic adenoma: 1 – normal colon mucosa, 2 – stalk of the polyp, 3 – tubulovillous colonic adenomatous polyp (Image courtesy of VE, used with permission).

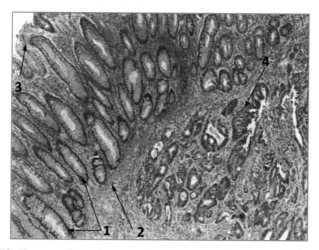

Figure 178. Hematoxylin and Eosin staining using 50 × objective of colon adenocarcinoma: 1 – colonic crypts lined by normal epithelium, 2 – muscularis mucosa, 3 – luminal surface of the mucosa lined by normal epithelium, 4 – adenocarcinoma of the colon invading the submucosa (Image courtesy of VE, used with permission).

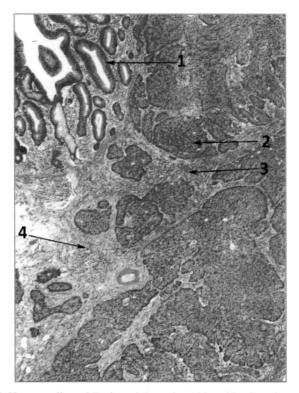

Figure 179. Hematoxylin and Eosin staining using 100 × objective of neuroendocrine carcinoma of the colon (2): 1 – tubulovillous adenoma of the colon, 3, 4 – peritumoral lymphocytic infiltrate (Image courtesy of VE, used with permission).

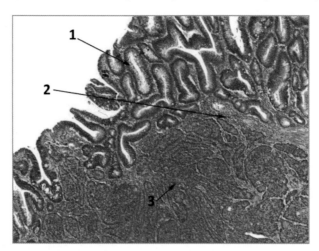

Figure 180. Hematoxylin and Eosin staining using 100 × objective of neuroendocrine carcinoma of the colon (3): 1 – tubulovillous adenoma of the colon, 2 – peritumoral lymphocytic infiltrate (Image courtesy of VE, used with permission).

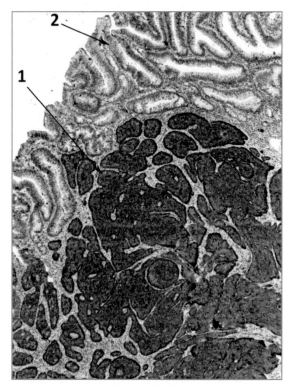

Figure 181. Immunohistochemistry expression of synaptophysin, using 100 × objective. Colon neuroendocrine tumor cells (1) showing immunoreactivity, while colon adenoma (2) tissue shows the absence of reactivity (Image courtesy of VE, used with permission).

The submucosa contains collagen and elastic fibers, local enteric nervous system (Meissner and Henle), vessels, lymphatic, inflammatory cells, and so on. Typically it is very loose, allowing the mucosal layer to glide over it during normal peristaltic movements.

The muscle layer contains an internal, circular and an external, longitudinal layer, with variable thickness depending on the colonic region. Between them is located the Auerbach's plexus and also interstitial Cajal cells.

SECTION XIV – THE RECTUM

To preserve and to renew is almost as noble as to create.

Voltaire

CHAPTER 40
EMBRYOLOGY

RUXANDRA IRINA NEGOI

The rectum and surgical anal canal above the dentate line receive their vascularization from the inferior mesenteric artery and veins, the main vessels of the hindgut. The lymphatic drainage is accomplished by the lymph nodes along these vessels. Innervation is provided by the autonomic nervous system (Negoi *et al.*, 2010).

The segment of the surgical anal canal below the dentate line has its embryological origin in the proctodeum, an ectodermal structure. According to this, this segment of the anal canal has a stratified squamous epithelium and receives its vascularization from the inferior rectal arteries, branches of the internal pudendal vessels. Lymphatic drainage is to the superficial inguinal lymph nodes. The innervation is from the somatic nervous system.

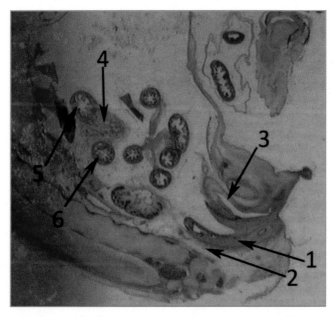

Figure 182. Sagittal section through the pelvis of a rat embryo revealing the rectum (1) with mesorectum (2), urinary bladder (3). Can be observed also, the pancreatic head (4), first (5) and third (6) duodenal segments (5) (Figure personal courtesy of RIN).

CHAPTER 41

ANATOMY

IONUȚ NEGOI, MIRCEA BEURAN

The upper limit of the rectum is at the third sacral vertebra, and the inferior limit is represented by the anal verge. Its length is 15 cm from the anal verge (Negoi *et al.*, 2010). The surgical anal canal has a length of 4 cm from the anal verge, while the anatomic anal canal is 2 cm long.

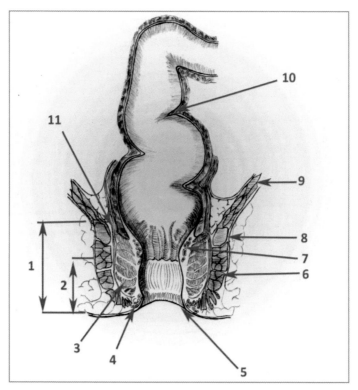

Figure 183. Schematic representation of a coronal section through the rectum: 1 – surgical anal canal, 2 – anatomical anal canal, 3 – internal anal sphincter, 4 – external hemorrhoidal plexus, 5 – anal verge, 6 – external anal sphincter, 7 – internal hemorrhoidal plexus, 8 – puborectalis muscle, 9 – levator ani muscle, 10 – superior valve of Houston (Image courtesy of IN).

From a surgical point of view, the rectum is divided into three segments:

Upper rectum: 11–15 cm from the anal verge, covered by peritoneum on its anterior and lateral sides.

Middle rectum 7–11 cm from the anal verge, covered by visceral peritoneum only on its anterior surface.

Lower rectum: 0–7 cm from the anal verge.

Measurement of rectal tumors from the anal verge should be done with a rigid proctosigmoidoscope and not with a flexible instrument which introduces an important degree of variability. Based on the local recurrence rate of rectal tumors, the National Cancer Institute establish the length of the rectum to be 12 cm above the anal verge (Nelson *et al.*, 2001).

CURVATURES

In the sagittal plane, the rectum presents two curvatures. The upper one has its concavity anteriorly, corresponding to the sacrum direction. The lower one is determined by the levator ani muscle and is concave posteriorly (the perineal curvature).

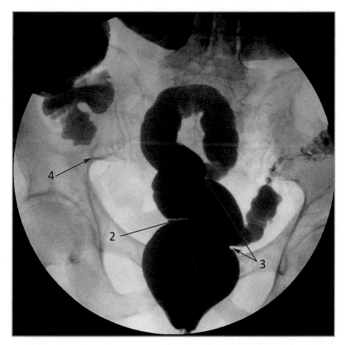

Figure 184. Barium enema revealing the rectum (1) with left (2) and rights (3) Houston valves, vermiform appendix (4) (Image from Collection of Radiology and Imagistics Department, Emergency Hospital of Bucharest).

In the coronal plane, the rectum has three curvatures which determine on its inside the valves of Houston.

These valves disappear after surgical circumferential mobilization of the rectum, the rectum elongates with a mean of 5 cm. According to this, a tumor located 6 cm from the anal verge will be found at 11 cm after circumferential mobilization of the rectum, in the mesorectal plane down to the levator ani muscles.

INTERNAL CONFIGURATION

ANAL CANAL

The anatomical anal canal is limited inferiorly by the anal verge and superiorly by the dentate line, with a length of two cm. The surgical anal canal is limited superiorly by the anorectal line, and is four cm long. The anatomical anal canal has an ectodermal embryological origin, similar to the skin. The rectum, above the dentate line, has an endodermal embryological origin, similar to the rest of the digestive tract. According to this the dentate line is an important boundary for its vascular supply, its lymphatic drainage and its innervation. The rectum narrows at the junction with the anal canal, determining the anal columns of Morgagni. The base of these columns are joined by anal valves. Above each anal valve is located a small pocket, termed an anal crypt. Inside these crypts are openings of the anal glands.

ANATOMICAL RELATIONSHIPS

RECTUM

The upper rectum is covered by peritoneum on its anterior and lateral surfaces. The middle rectum is covered by visceral peritoneum only on its anterior surface, while the inferior rectum is totally extraperitoneal.

Above the peritoneal reflection

Anteriorly: the ileal loops and the sigmoid colon, the fundus of the urinary bladder (in males), posterior surface of the uterus, the fallopian tubes, the ovaries and the posterior vaginal wall (in females).

Laterally: the peritoneum reflects on the lateral pelvic sidewalls giving rise to the pararectal fossa.

Below the peritoneal reflection

Anteriorly, in males: Denonvilliers' fascia, the prostate, the seminal vesicles, the deferent ducts, the ureters and the fundus of the urinary bladder. In females: the recto-vaginal septum and the posterior vaginal wall.

Laterally: the inferior hypogastric plexuses.

Posteriorly: the presacral fascia, the middle sacral and lateral sacral vessels, the sacral sympathetic chains and sacral spinal nerves.

The subperitoneal rectum is surrounded by fatty tissue termed the mesorectum, widely popularized in the last 25 years by B. Heald. The mesorectum is wrapped in the mesorectal fascia, or the fascia propria of the rectum. Inside the mesorectum are located terminal braches of the superior rectal artery and vein, together with the regional lymph nodes (Negoi *et al.*, 2010).

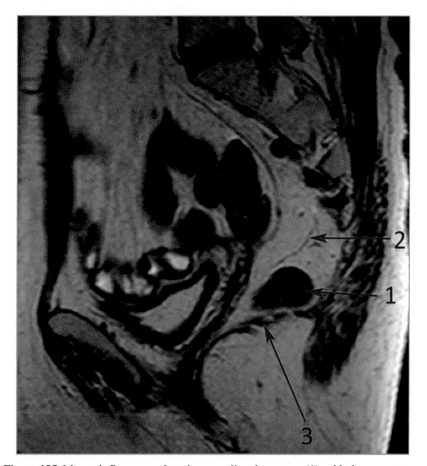

Figure 185. Magnetic Resonance Imaging revealing the rectum (1), with the mesorectum including branches of the superior rectal vessels (2), and levator ani muscles (3) (Image courtesy of Radiology and Imagistics Department, Emergency Hospital of Bucharest).

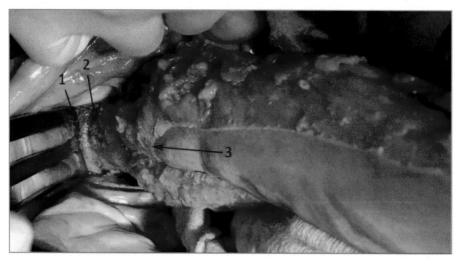

Figure 186. Intraoperative view of the surgical dissection into the anterior aspect of the "holly plane" during an open low anterior resection of the rectum: 1 – posterior wall of the vagina, 2 – anterior mesorectum, significantly thinner in this point, 3 – incised peritoneum at the level of the Douglas pouch (Image courtesy of IN).

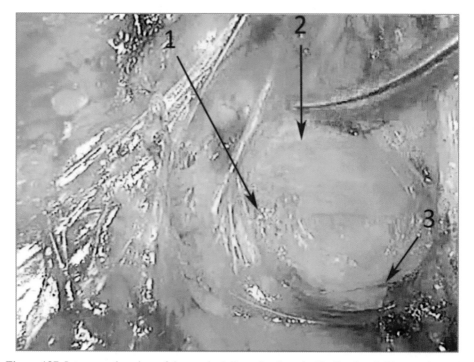

Figure 187. Intraoperative view of the surgical dissection into the "holly plane" (1) posterior to the mesorectal fascia (2) and anterior to the presacral fascia (3) during a laparoscopic low anterior resection of the rectum (Image courtesy of SP, used with permission).

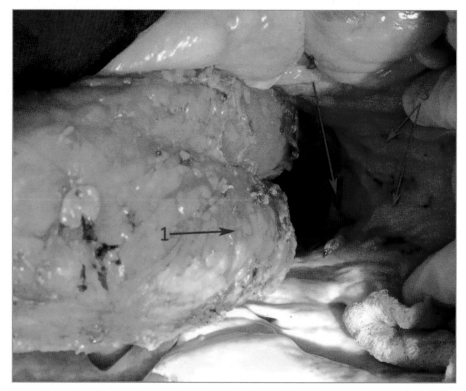

Figure 188. Intraoperative view of the surgical dissection into the "holly plane" posterior to the mesorectal fascia (1) and anterior to the presacral fascia (2) during an open low anterior resection of the rectum. 3 – the two hypogastric nerves (Image courtesy of IN).

ANAL CANAL

Anteriorly:

Male: the prostate, the membranous urethra, the deep transverse muscle of the perineum, the bulb of the penis, and the tendinous center of the perineum.

Female: the lower segment of the vagina and the tendinous center of the perineum.

Posteriorly: the anococcygeal ligament.

Laterally: the ischioanal fossa.

The ischioanal fossa is a pyramidal space, with the following boundaries: (a) Laterally – the internal obturator muscle; (b) Medially – the external anal sphincter; (c) superior and medial – the levator ani muscle; (d) inferiorly – the perineal skin.

On the lateral wall of the ischioanal fossa, in the fascia of the internal obturator muscle, is located the pudendal canal of Alcock. This canal includes the internal pudendal artery, vein and nerve (Negoi *et al.*, 2010).

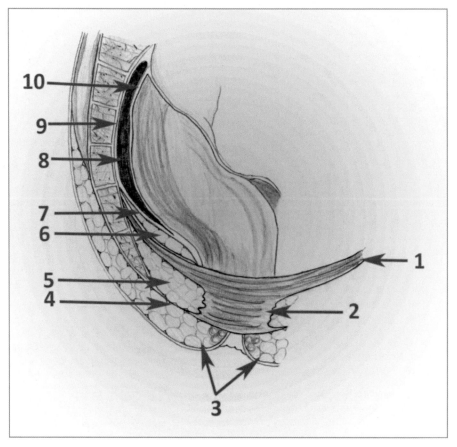

Figure 189. Schematic representation of a coronal section through the rectum: 1 – levator ani muscle, 2 – external anal sphincter, 3 – perianal space, 4 – anococcygeal ligament, 5 – deep postanal space, 6 – supralevator retrorectal space, 7 – rectosacral fascia, 8 – mesorectum, 9 – presacral fascia, 10 – mesorectal fascia [Image redrawn by IN from Wexner *et al.* (Wexner and Jorge, 2005).

VASCULAR SUPPLY

ARTERIES

Arterial blood supply of the rectum is accomplished by the upper, middle and inferior rectal arteries. The superior rectal artery continues the trajectory of the inferior mesenteric artery. It descends through the sigmoid mesocolon, crosses the common iliac vessels and enters the mesorectum. At the level of the third sacral vertebra, inside the mesorectum, the superior rectal artery branches off into a right and left branch.

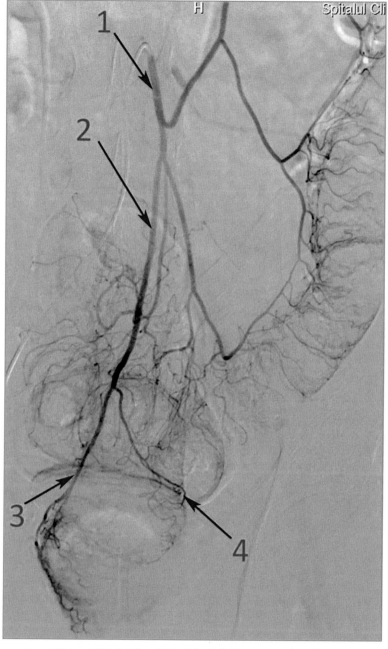

Figure 190. Angiography of the inferior mesenteric artery
(1) revealing the superior rectal artery (2) with its right (3) and left branches
(4) (Figure courtesy of Emergency Hospital of Bucharest,
Department of Angiography).

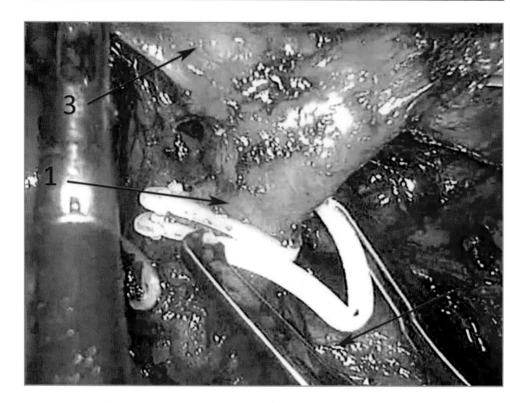

Figure 191. Intraoperative view of the inferior mesenteric artery (1) at its emergence
from the aorta (2), clipped above the emergence of left colic artery (3) during a
laparoscopic low anterior resection of the rectum (Image courtesy of IN).

There they divide into smaller branches, which traverse the muscularis
propria of the rectum, reaching the submucosal network. In the rectal submucosa,
the terminal branches of the superior rectal artery anastomose with the inferior
rectal artery. The middle rectal artery emerges from the internal iliac artery, usually
through a common trunk with the inferior vesical or uterine artery. Bill Heald
observed that if the rectal dissection is done in the correct plane, the mesorectal
one, the surgeon will find laterally only a small artery, which requires only a small
touch with the electrocautery. The middle rectal artery was found with a frequency
of 12% on both sides and in 22% unilaterally (Ayoub, 1978; Heald and Moran,
1998).

The inferior rectal artery is a branch of the internal pudendal artery, in
Alcock's canal. From its origin it has a transverse course, in the ischioanal fossa.
Traversing the external anal sphincter, ending in the submucosal network of the
rectum.

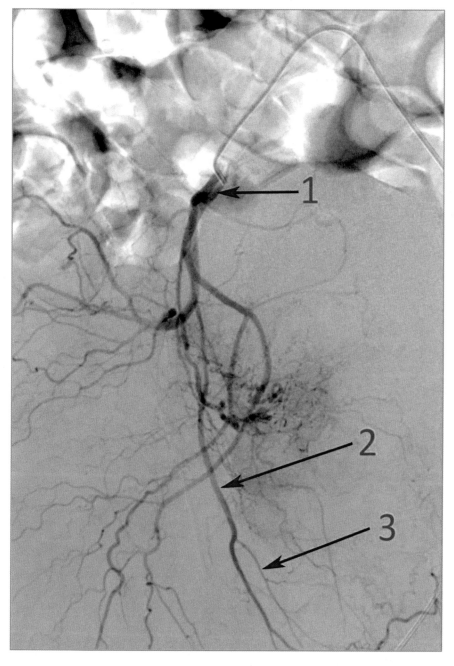

Figure 192. Angiography of right internal iliac artery (1) revealing the internal pudendal artery (2) with the inferior rectal artery (3) (Figure courtesy of Emergency Hospital of Bucharest, Department of Angiography).

VEINS

The venous drainage of the rectum is superposed to its arterial supply, with a superior, middle and inferior rectal vein. The superior rectal vein drains into the inferior mesenteric vein, the middle rectal vein drains into the internal iliac vein and from here into the common iliac and the inferior vena cava. The inferior rectal veins drain into the internal pudendal vein, into the internal and common iliac and from here into the inferior vena cava.

All these veins drain the rectum, which has two venous plexuses:
- internal rectal plexus (located in the submucosa).
- external rectal plexus, perirectal or perimuscular (located outside the muscularis propria).

The internal rectal plexus, located in the submucosa, is divided by the dentate line in the internal hemorrhoidal plexus (located above) and external hemorrhoidal plexus (located below).

"Corpus cavernosum recti"

In the submucosa of the surgical anal canal is located an arteriovenous anastomosis best described as "corpus cavernosum rectum". The superior rectal artery terminal branches end in the corpus cavernosum rectum, while the drainage is through superior, middle and inferior rectal veins. The morphology of this anorectal vascular plexus seems to be similar with the penile corpus cavernosum. The venous capillaries at this level have a similar glomerular anatomy, with the sphincters that regulate blood filling and draining. Impairment of the balance between blood inflow and outflow, is the key factor in the pathogenesis of hemorrhoids.

LYMPHATICS

The rectum has a very rich lymphatic network in the submucosa. Lymphatic capillaries penetrate the muscularis propria of the rectum, and from there the drainage occurs further into the epirectal and pararectal lymph nodes, located into the mesorectum. Canessa *et al.* found through anatomical dissection a mean of 8.4 lymph nodes in the mesorectum. Using chemical methods, other researchers revealed 73.7 lymph nodes inside the mesorectum (Canessa *et al.*, 2001). 71.4% of lymph nodes were located around the branches of the superior rectal artery, proximal to the peritoneal reflection, and 28.6% were found distal to the peritoneal reflection (Canessa *et al.*, 2001). The epirectal lymphnodes are termed Gerota's nodes (Wexner and Jorge, 2005).

The dentate line represents the watershed between two lymphatic territories:

Above the dentate line the lymphatic drainage is toward the inferior mesenteric lymph nodes.

Below the dentate line the lymphatic drainage is toward the superficial inguinal lymph nodes.

The lymph of the upper and middle rectum drains into the superior rectal lymph nodes and from here into the inferior mesenteric lymph nodes. The lower rectum drains into the superior rectal and inferior mesenteric lymph nodes, but also through the middle rectal lymphatics into the internal iliac lymph nodes. According to Stelzner, the lymphatic drainage of the rectum is toward the inferior mesenteric lymph nodes, the lymphatic vessels present unidirectional valves which prevents reflux of the lymph (Stelzner, 2007). The lymphatic vessels located around the middle rectal vessels are scarce, with rare lymph node metastasis of rectal cancer into the internal iliac lymph nodes. Considering that the lymphatic spread of rectal cancer is to the lymph nodes located above and below the levator ani muscles, Miles recommended abdominoperineal resection as a radical approach to rectal cancer. Bill Heald disagreed with this concept, he considers that the lymphatic drainage of the rectum is only above the levator ani muscle, and that the majority of rectal cancers can be managed by a sphincter saving procedure (Heald and Moran, 1998).

INNERVATION

The innervation of the rectum above the dentate line is autonomous, from the inferior mesenteric periarterial plexus. The anatomical anal canal receives its somatic innervation through the inferior rectal nerve, a branch of the internal pudendal nerve. The traditional approach to rectal cancer was followed by sexual and urinary dysfunctions. Following Bill Heald's concept of total mesorectal excision in 1979, Enker proposed in 1991 total mesorectal excision with autonomic nerve preservation (Havenga and Enker, 2002). Superior hypogastric plexus is represented by a nervous network located anterior to the aortic bifurcation and sacral promontorium and medial to the common iliac arteries. This plexus includes only sympathetic fibers, which come from the preaortic plexus (located above) and from the lumbar nerves. The superior hypogastric plexus is continued downward with the hypogastric nerves.

The hypogastric nerves, which include only sympathetic fibers, are located 1 cm lateral to the promontorium, then have a descending trajectory, 1–2 cm medial to the ureters (Nivatvongs and Gordon, 2007). At the level of the pelvic sidewalls, the hypogastric nerves end in the inferior hypogastric plexus. The operating surgeon should note that the hypogastric nerves are outside the mesorectal fascia, and medial to the parietal pelvic fascia. They adhere to the mesorectal fascia, and should be carefully lateralized during surgical dissection, preventing their injury (Heald, 2007).

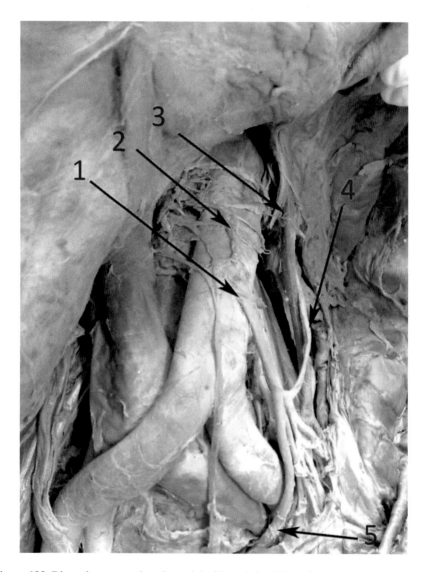

Figure 193. Dissection on a cadaveric model of the origin of the inferior mesenteric artery (1), the preaortic nervous plexus (2), inferior mesenteric vein (3), left colic artery (4), and superior rectal artery (5) (Image courtesy of IN).

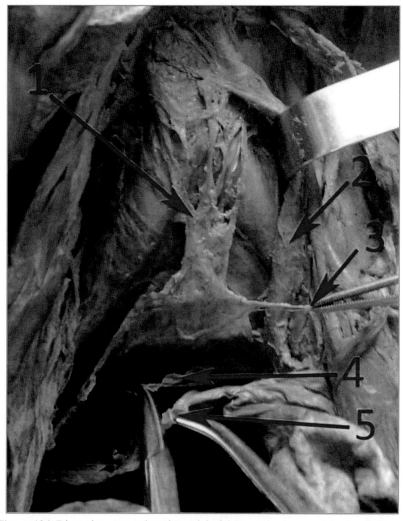

Figure 194. Dissection on a cadaveric model of the superior hypogastric plexus (1) and the two hypogastric nerves (3). 2 – superior rectal artery, 4 – mesorectal fascia, 5 – peritoneum of the Douglas pouch (Image courtesy of IN).

The inferior hypogastric plexus is a nervous network, with a semi-sagittal orientation, between the mesorectal fascia and the parietal endopelvic fascia (Takahashi *et al.*, 2000). It is 4 – 5 cm in length, is crossed by arteries and veins which supply the rectum, urinary bladder and internal genitalia. The inferior hypogastric plexus is continued anteriorly by neurovascular bundles of Walsh, located at the level of the prostate in a 5 and 7 o'clock position. The inferior hypogastric plexus receives sympathetic fibers from the hypogastric nerves and parasympathetic fibers from the erector nerves. The erector nerves, or the pelvic splanchnic nerves have their origin in the second, third and fourth sacral spinal cord.

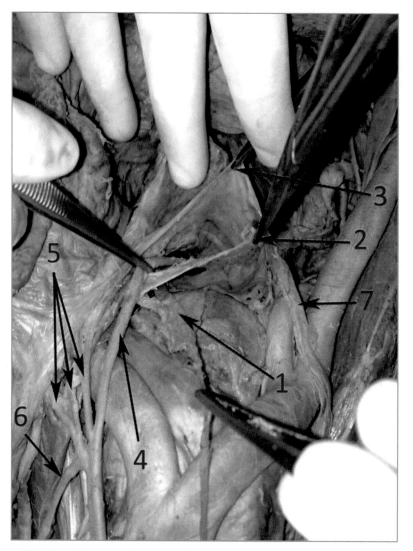

Figure 195. Dissection on a cadaveric model of the left hypogastric nerve with its trajectory outside the mesorectal fascia (2) but anterior to the presacral fascia (posterior parietal pelvic fascia). 3 – peritoneum of the Douglas pouch, 4 – superior rectal artery entering the mesorectum, 5 – sigmoidian arteries, 6 – left colic artery, 7 – right ureter (Image courtesy of IN).

MESORECTUM

Although used in medical literature for over 100 years, the term "mesorectum" was widely popularized by Bill Heald, from Basingstoke District Hospital, United Kingdom.

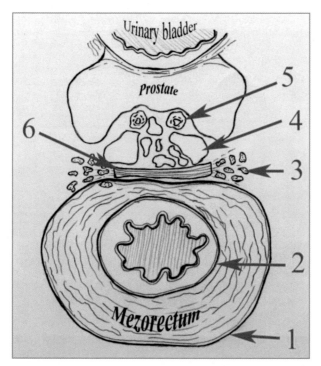

Figure 196. Schematic representation of the mesorectum: 1 – mesorectal fascia, 2 – muscularis propria of rectum, 3 – neuromuscular bundles of Walsh, 4 – seminal vesicles, 5 – duct deferens, 6 – Denonvillier fascia (Image courtesy of IN).

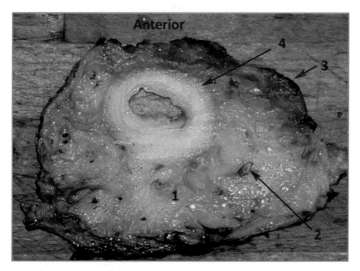

Figure 197. Transverse section through the rectum and mesorectum. 1 – mesorectum, 2 – arterial branch from the superior rectal artery inside the mesorectum, 3 – mesorectal fascia, 4 – muscularis propria of the rectum (Image courtesy of VE, used with permission).

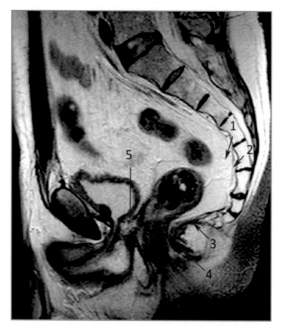

Figure 198. Magnetic Resonance Imaging revealing the mesorectum(1), enclosed by the mesorectal fascia (2). 3 – levator ani muscle, 4 – external anal sphincter muscle, 5 – prostate (Image courtesy of Radiology and Imagistics Department, Emergency Hospital of Bucharest).

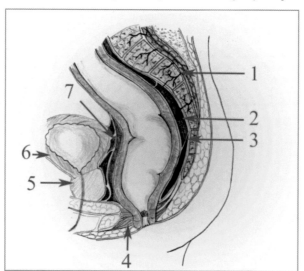

Figure 199. Schematic representation of a coronal section through the rectum: 1 – basivertebral plexus which bleeds massively during surgical dissection posterior to the presacral fascia, 2 – mesorectum, 3 – rectosacral fascia located between presacral fascia and mesorectal fascia (during surgical dissection into the mesorectal plane it should be divided, blunt dissection tearing the mesorectal fascia and not this anatomical resistant structure), 4 – external anal sphincter, 5 – prostate, 6 – urinary bladder (Image courtesy of IN).

Although not a mesentery according to the classical definition, the mesorectum represents a visceral package which includes the terminal branches of the inferior mesenteric artery, the veins tributaries to the inferior mesenteric vein, and lymphatics, all these structures being surrounded by visceral fat and covered by a clearly identifiable mesorectal fascia (Chapuis *et al.*, 2002).

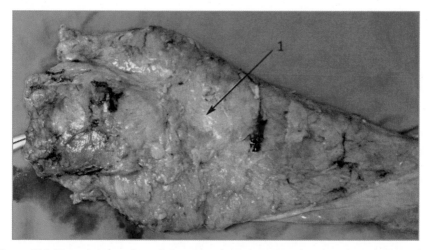

Figure 200. Intraoperative view of the resected specimen in a low anterior resection of the rectum with total mesorectal excision for a middle rectal cancer. It can be observed the integrity of the shiny fascial structure surrounding the mesorectum, termed mesorectal fascia (Image from personal collection of IN).

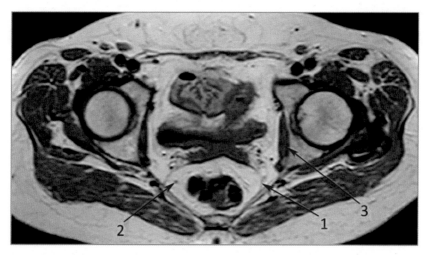

Figure 201. Magnetic Resonance Imaging revealing the mesorectum enclosed by the mesorectal fascia (1): 2 – branches of the superior rectal vessels included in the mesorectum, 3 – internal obturator muscle (Image courtesy of Radiology and Imagistics Department, Emergency Hospital of Bucharest).

On MRI the mesorectum appears as an adipose envelope, with hyposignal for vessels and hypersignal for lymph nodes. The preoperative staging of patients with rectal cancer, is accomplished with fine slice MRI should establish the distance between the tumor and the mesorectal fascia. Whenever this fascia is threatened, the tumor should be downstaged and downsized by neoadjuvant chemoradiation.

According to Heald, a high quality surgical specimen, should present the following characteristics (Heald, 2007):

On its anterior surface: the incised peritoneum (upper part), the shiny and smooth Denonvillier's or rectovaginal fascia (middle part).

Lateral and posterior: an intact mesorectal fascia, which presents in the caudal part an anteroposterior groove, determined by the inferior hypogastric plexus.

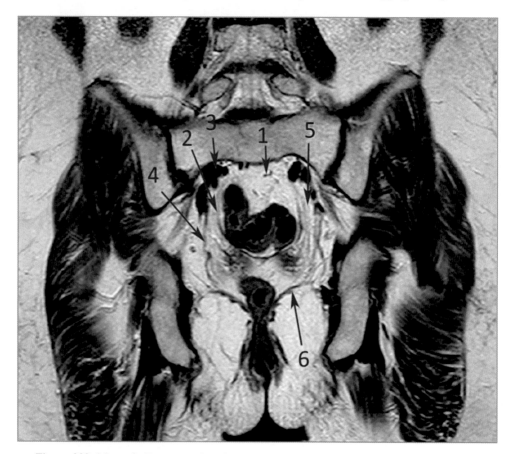

Figure 202. Magnetic Resonance Imaging, coronal section, revealing the vessels inside the mesorectum (1), mesorectal fascia (2), internal iliac vessels (3) with their emerging vessels (4), internal hypogastric plexus (5) and levator ani muscle (6) (Image courtesy of Radiology and Imagistics Department, Emergency Hospital of Bucharest).

EXTRALEVATOR ABDOMINOPERINEAL RESECTION
FOR LOW RECTAL CANCER

Recent evidence proved that conventional abdominoperineal resection (CAPR) for low rectal cancer was associated with an increased rate of positive circumferential resection margin (CRM) and intraoperative tumor perforation than anterior resection for stage-matched tumors located high in the rectum (Law and Chu, 2004; Nagtegaal *et al.*, 2005; den Dulk *et al.*, 2009). This seems to be a consequence of a "waisted" specimen after CAPR, where abdominal and perineal dissections meet (Holm *et al.*, 2007). In an effort to improve the quality of the resected specimen and the long-term oncological outcomes, the European surgeons proposed a more extensive extralevator dissection, termed extralevator abdominoperineal excision (ELAPE) (Holm *et al.*, 2007; West *et al.*, 2010b). In fact, ELAPE is a return to Miles' original technique, which recommended division of the levators "as far outwards as their origin from the white line so as to include the lateral zone of spread" (Miles). For a cylindrical specimen, during ELAPE the mesorectum is not dissected off the levators during abdominal phase, with en bloc excision of the levators during perineal phase (Ramsay *et al.*, 2013). While CAPR is performed in a lithotomy position, the ELAPE is performed in the prone jackknife position, which allows a more anatomical perineal surgical dissection (Liu *et al.*, 2015).

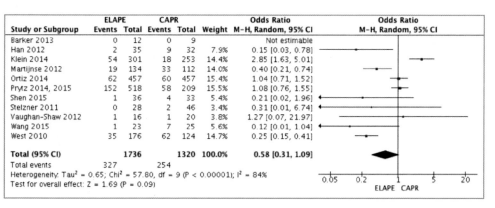

Figure 203. Meta-analysis of studies on circumferential resection margin involvement of patients undergoing extralevator abdominoperineal excision (ELAPE) *versus* conventional abdominoperineal excision (CAPR) (Negoi *et al.*, 2015b).

There are four recent systematic reviews and meta-analysis (Yu *et al.*, 2014; Huang *et al.*, 2014b; De Nardi *et al.*, 2015; Zhou *et al.*, 2015) comparing the conventional with the extralevator abdominoperineal resection with contradictory results, three claiming superiority (Yu *et al.*, 2014; Huang *et al.*, 2014b; De Nardi *et al.*, 2015) and one the equivalence (Zhou *et al.*, 2015) of ELAPE concerning CRM positivity and intraoperative perforation rate. On the other hand, during the last three years there have been published, four high quality studies which question the benefits of ELAPE as a standard procedure (Krishna *et al.*, 2013; Ortiz *et al.*, 2014; Prytz *et al.*, 2015; Klein *et al.*, 2015).

A systematic review and meta-analysis performed by the authors of this book included in total one Randomized Control Trial and ten non-randomized comparative studies, involving 1736 patients in the ELAPE group and 1320 patients in the CAPR group (Negoi *et al.*, 2015b). The ELAPE was associated with a significantly lower intraoperative perforation rate. There were no differences regarding the circumferential margin involvement, R0 resections and local recurrence rate.

CHAPTER 42

HISTOLOGY

VALENTIN ENACHE, SORIN HOSTIUC

The anatomical anal canal, two cm long, has its mucosal layer tapered with squamous cell stratified epithelium. Above the dentate line, the rectum has its mucosa layer tapered with columnar unistratified epithelium.

Compared to the other structures of the lower gastrointestinal system, the anal canal is more complex.

The epithelium is separated into four main areas:

• The most internal part is covered by uninterrupted mucosa similar to that from the colon. There is no clearly distinct area of separation from the colon, but are identifiable crypts that are more irregular compared to the normal structure of the colon.

• Next is an area called the anal transitional zone, containing epithelial cells appertaining to both colon and squamous area.

• Next is an area covered by unkeratinized squamous epithelium. It doesn't contain papillae, glands, or skin appendages, but are identifiable Langerhans, T lymphocytes and Merkel cells.

• Last is an area covered by keratinized squamous epithelium and skin appendages. In this area are easily identifiable glands (sebaceous, sweat), and hair follicles.

BIBLIOGRAPHY

Abdalla EK., Vauthey J-N., Couinaud C. 2002. The caudate lobe of the liver: implications of embryology and anatomy for surgery. *Surgical oncology clinics of North America* 11:835–48.

Abdel-Misih SRZ., Bloomston M. 2010. Liver anatomy. *The Surgical clinics of North America* 90:643–53.

Adham M., Singhirunnusorn J. 2012. Surgical technique and results of total mesopancreas excision (TMpE) in pancreatic tumors. *European Journal of Surgical Oncology: the Journal of the European Society of Surgical Oncology and the British Association of Surgical Oncology* 38:340–345.

Agrawal MK., Thakur DS., Somashekar U., Chandrakar SK., Sharma D. 2010. Mesopancreas: myth or reality? *JOP: Journal of the Pancreas* 11:230–233.

Akiyama H., Tsurumaru M., Kawamura T., Ono Y. 1981. Principles of surgical treatment for carcinoma of the esophagus: analysis of lymph node involvement. *Annals of Surgery* 194:438–46.

Akiyama H., Tsurumaru M., Ono Y., Udagawa H. KY. 1991. Background of Lymph Node Dissection for Squamous Cell Carcinoma of the Esophagus. In: Sato. T, Iizuka T eds. *Color Atlas of Surgical Anatomy for Esophageal Cancer.* Springer-Verlag, 9–24.

Albanese AM., Albanese EF., Miño JH., Gómez E., Gómez M., Zandomeni M., Merlo AB. 2009. Peritoneal surface area: measurements of 40 structures covered by peritoneum: correlation between total peritoneal surface area and the surface calculated by formulas. *Surgical and Radiologic Anatomy: SRA* 31:369–77.

Alexakis N., Halloran C., Raraty M., Ghaneh P., Sutton R., Neoptolemos JP. 2004. Current standards of surgery for pancreatic cancer. *British Journal of Surgery* 91:1410–1427.

Ayoub SF. 1978. Arterial supply to the human rectum. *Cells Tissues Organs* 100:317–327.

Ba-Ssalamah A., Bastati N., Uffmann M., Pretterklieber M., Schima W. 2009. [Peritoneum and mesenterium. Radiological anatomy and extent of peritoneal diseases]. *Der Radiologe* 49:543–54; quiz 555–6.

Baque P., Iannelli A., Delotte J., de Peretti F., Bourgeon A. 2009. Division of the right posterior attachments of the head of the pancreas with a linear stapler during pancreaticoduodenectomy: vascular and oncological considerations based on an anatomical cadaver-based study. *Surgical and Radiologic Anatomy: SRA* 31:13–17.

Benacci JC., Deschamps C., Trastek VF., Allen MS., Daly RC., Pairolero PC. 1993. Epiphrenic diverticulum: results of surgical treatment. *The Annals of Thoracic Surgery* 55:1109–1113; discussion 1114.

Beuran M., Negoi I., Paun S., Ion AD., Bleotu C., Negoi RI., Hostiuc S. 2015. The epithelial to mesenchymal transition in pancreatic cancer: A systematic review. *Pancreatology: Official Journal of the International Association of Pancreatology (IAP) ... [et al.]* 15:217–25.

Bismuth H., Houssin D., Castaing D. 1982. Major and minor segmentectomies "réglées" in liver surgery. *World Journal of Surgery* 6:10–24.

Blackburn SC., Stanton MP. 2014. Anatomy and physiology of the peritoneum. *Seminars in Pediatric Surgery* 23:326–30.

Bonenkamp JJ., Songun I., Hermans J., Sasako M., Welvaart K., Plukker JT., van Elk P., Obertop H., Gouma DJ., Taat CW. 1995. Randomised comparison of morbidity after D1 and D2 dissection for gastric cancer in 996 Dutch patients. *Lancet (London, England)* 345:745–8.

Broering D., Walter J., Halata Z. 2009. Surgical Anatomy of the Esophagus. In: Izbicki J, Broering D, Yekebas E, Kutup A, Chernousov A, N. YIGPMB eds. *Surgery of the Esophagus: Textbook and Atlas of Surgical Practice.* Steinkopff Verlag, 3–9.

Brown TH., Davidson PF., Larson GM. 1989. Acute gastritis occurring within 24 hours of severe head injury. *Gastrointestinal Endoscopy* 35:37–40.

Cameron AJ., Lomboy CT., Pera M., Carpenter HA. 1995. Adenocarcinoma of the esophagogastric junction and Barrett's esophagus. *Gastroenterology* 109:1541–1546.

Canessa CE., Badía F., Fierro S., Fiol V., Háyek G. 2001. Anatomic study of the lymph nodes of the mesorectum. *Diseases of the Colon and Rectum* 44:1333–6.

Castaing D. 2008. Surgical anatomy of the biliary tract. *HPB: The Official Journal of the International Hepato Pancreato Biliary Association* 10:72–6.

Chapuis P., Bokey L., Fahrer M., Sinclair G., Bogduk N. 2002. Mobilization of the rectum: anatomic concepts and the bookshelf revisited. *Diseases of the Colon and Rectum* 45:1–8; discussion 8–9.

Cho A., Yamamoto H., Kainuma O. 2014. Tips of laparoscopic pancreaticoduodenectomy: superior mesenteric artery first approach (with video). *Journal of Hepato-Biliary-Pancreatic Sciences* 21:E19–E21.

Choi YY., An JY., Guner A., Kang DR., Cho I., Kwon IG., Shin HB., Hyung WJ., Noh SH. 2015. Skip lymph node metastasis in gastric cancer: is it skipping or skipped? *Gastric Cancer: Official Journal of the International Gastric Cancer Association and the Japanese Gastric Cancer Association.*

Clark SB., Rice TW., Tubbs RR., Richter JE., Goldblum JR. 2000. The nature of the myenteric infiltrate in achalasia: an immunohistochemical analysis. *The American Journal of Surgical Pathology* 24:1153–8.

Correa P. 1988. Chronic gastritis: a clinico-pathological classification. *The American Journal of Gastroenterology* 83:504–9.

Couinaud C. 1957. *Le Foi: Études Anatomogiques et Chirurgicales.* Masson Paris.

Couinaud C. 1999. Liver anatomy: portal (and suprahepatic) or biliary segmentation. *Digestive Surgery* 16:459–67.

Cullen JM. 2005. Mechanistic classification of liver injury. *Toxicologic Pathology* 33:6–8.

Cuschieri A., Fayers P., Fielding J., Craven J., Bancewicz J., Joypaul V., Cook P. 1996. Postoperative morbidity and mortality after D1 and D2 resections for gastric cancer: preliminary results of the MRC randomised controlled surgical trial. The Surgical Cooperative Group. *Lancet (London, England)* 347:995–9.

Cuschieri A., Weeden S., Fielding J., Bancewicz J., Craven J., Joypaul V., Sydes M., Fayers P. 1999. Patient survival after D1 and D2 resections for gastric cancer: long-term results of the MRC randomized surgical trial. Surgical Co-operative Group. *British Journal of Cancer* 79:1522–30.

Dahmane R., Morjane A., Ravnik D., Hribernik M. 2009. Anatomy of the ligamentum venosum arantii and its contribution to the left hepatic vein and common trunk control. A study on cadaveric livers. *Cells, Tissues, Organs* 190:297–300.

Degiuli M., Sasako M., Ponti A., Vendrame A., Tomatis M., Mazza C., Borasi A., Capussotti L., Fronda G., Morino M. 2014. Randomized clinical trial comparing survival after D1 or D2 gastrectomy for gastric cancer. *The British Journal of Surgery* 101:23–31.

Degiuli M., Sasako M., Ponti A. 2010. Morbidity and mortality in the Italian Gastric Cancer Study Group randomized clinical trial of D1 versus D2 resection for gastric cancer. *The British Journal of Surgery* 97:643–9.

Delis KT., Gloviczki P., Altuwaijri M., McKusick MA. 2007. Median arcuate ligament syndrome: open celiac artery reconstruction and ligament division after endovascular failure. *Journal of Vascular Surgery* 46:799–802.

Delpero JR., Bachellier P., Regenet N., Le Treut YP., Paye F., Carrere N., Sauvanet A., Autret A., Turrini O., Monges-Ranchin G., Boher JM. 2014. Pancreaticoduodenectomy for pancreatic ductal adenocarcinoma: a French multicentre prospective evaluation of resection margins in 150 evaluable specimens. *HPB: The Official Journal of the International Hepato Pancreato Biliary Association* 16:20–33.

Dodds WJ., Dent J., Hogan WJ., Helm JF., Hauser R., Patel GK., Egide MS. 1982. Mechanisms of gastroesophageal reflux in patients with reflux esophagitis. *The New England Journal of Medicine* 307:1547–52.

den Dulk M., Putter H., Collette L., Marijnen CAM., Folkesson J., Bosset J-F., Rödel C., Bujko K., Påhlman L., van de Velde CJH. 2009. The abdominoperineal resection itself is associated with an adverse outcome: the European experience based on a pooled analysis of five European randomised clinical trials on rectal cancer. *European Journal of Cancer (Oxford, England: 1990)* 45:1175–83.

Edge S., Byrd DR., Compton CC., Fritz AG., Greene FL., Trotti A. 2010. *AJCC Cancer Staging Manual*. Springer.

Ellis FH., Schlegel JF., Lynch VP., Payne WS. 1969. Cricopharyngeal myotomy for pharyngoesophageal diverticulum. *Annals of Surgery* 170:340–9.

Endo T., Arimura Y., Adachi Y., Mita H., Yamashita K., Yamamoto H., Shinomura Y., Ishii Y. 2012. A case of Ménétrier's disease without Helicobacter pylori infection. *Digestive endoscopy: Official Journal of the Japan Gastroenterological Endoscopy Society* 24:275–9.

Esposito I., Kleeff J., Bergmann F., Reiser C., Herpel E., Friess H., et a. l. 2008. Most pancreatic cancer resections are R1 resections. *Annals of Surgical Oncology* 15:1651–1660.

Evans DB., Pisters PW. 2003. Novel applications of endo GIA linear staplers during pancreaticoduodenectomy and total pancreatectomy. *American Journal of Surgery* 185:606–607.

Faitot F., Vibert E., Salloum C., Gorden DL., Coscas F., Adam R., Castaing D. 2012. Importance of conserving middle hepatic vein distal branches for homogeneous regeneration of the left liver after right hepatectomy. *HPB: the official journal of the International Hepato Pancreato Biliary Association* 14:746–53.

Gaedcke J., Gunawan B., Grade M., Szoke R., Liersch T., Becker H., et al. 2010. The mesopancreas is the primary site for R1 resection in pancreatic head cancer: relevance for clinical trials. *Langenbeck's Archives of Surgery / Deutsche Gesellschaft fur Chirurgie* 395:451–458.

Gertler R., Rosenberg R., Feith M., Schuster T., Friess H. 2009. Pouch vs. no pouch following total gastrectomy: meta-analysis and systematic review. *The American Journal of Gastroenterology* 104:2838–51.

Goldsmith, N.A., Woodburne RT. 1957. The surgical anatomy pertaining to liver resection. *Surgery, Gynecology and Obstetrics* 105:310–318.

Guglielmi A., Ruzzenente A., Iacono C. 2008. Surgical Anatomy of the Hepatic Hilus. In: *Surgical Treatment of Hilar and Intrahepatic Cholangiocarcinoma*. Springer, 101–113.

Hackert T., Weitz J., Büchler MW. 2015. Reinsertion of the gastric coronary vein to avoid venous gastric congestion in pancreatic surgery. *HPB: The Official Journal of the International Hepato Pancreato Biliary Association* 17:368–70.

Hann LE. 2012. *Blumgart's Surgery of the Liver, Pancreas and Biliary Tract*. Elsevier.

Hartgrink HH., van de Velde CJH., Putter H., Bonenkamp JJ., Klein Kranenbarg E., Songun I., Welvaart K., van Krieken JHJM., Meijer S., Plukker JTM., van Elk PJ., Obertop H., Gouma DJ., van Lanschot JJB., Taat CW., de Graaf PW., von Meyenfeldt MF., Tilanus H., Sasako M. 2004. Extended lymph node dissection for gastric cancer: who may benefit? Final results of the randomized Dutch gastric cancer group trial. *Journal of Clinical Oncology: Official Journal of the American Society of Clinical Oncology* 22:2069–77.

Hartley M., Finch-Jones M. 2003. Surgical anatomy of the pancreas. In: Poston G, Blumgart LH eds. *Surgical Management of Hepatobiliary and Pancreatic Disorders*. Martin Dunitz Ltd, a member of the Taylor and Francis group, 30–45.

Havenga K., Enker WE. 2002. Autonomic nerve preserving total mesorectal excision. *The Surgical Clinics of North America* 82:1009–18.

Heald R. 2007. Rectal Cancer in the 21st Century- radical Operations: anterior Resection and Abdominoperineal excision. In: Fischer J ed. *Mastery of Surgery*. Lippincott Williams and Wilkins, 1542–1555.

Heald RJ., Moran BJ. 1998. Embryology and anatomy of the rectum. *Seminars in Surgical Oncology* 15:66–71.

Healey, J.E., Schroy PC. 1953. Anatomy of the biliary ducts within the human liver. *Arch Surg* 66:599–616.

Hiatt JR., Gabbay J., Busuttil RW. 1994. Surgical anatomy of the hepatic arteries in 1000 cases. *Annals of Surgery* 220:50–2.

Higuchi T., Sugihara K. 2010. Complete mesocolic excision (CME) with central vascular ligation (CVL) as standardised surgical technique for colonic cancer: A Japanese multicentre study. *Dis Colon Rectum* 53:646.

Hirschfield G., Karlsen T., Lindor K., Adams D. 2013. Primary sclerosing cholangitis. *The Lancet.*

Hohenberger W., Weber K., Matzel K., Papadopoulos T., Merkel S. 2009. Standardized surgery for colonic cancer: Complete mesocolic excision and central ligation - Technical notes and outcome. *Colorectal Disease* 11:354–364.

Hohenberger W., Merkel S., Weber K. 2007. [Lymphadenectomy with tumors of the lower gastro-intestinal tract]. *Der Chirurg; Zeitschrift für alle Gebiete der operativen Medizen* 78:217–25.

Holm T., Ljung A., Häggmark T., Jurell G., Lagergren J. 2007. Extended abdominoperineal resection with gluteus maximus flap reconstruction of the pelvic floor for rectal cancer. *The British Journal of Surgery* 94:232–8.

Hruban R., Pitman M., Klimstra D. 2007. *Tumors of the Pancreas.*

Huang C-M., Chen Q-Y., Lin J-X., Zheng C-H., Li P., Xie J-W., Wang J-B., Lu J. 2013. Short-term clinical implications of the accessory left hepatic artery in patients undergoing radical gastrectomy for gastric cancer. *PloS one* 8:e64300.

Huang C-M., Wang J-B., Wang Y., Zheng C-H., Li P., Xie J-W., Lin J-X., Lu J. 2014a. Left gastric vein on the dorsal side of the splenic artery: a rare anatomic variant revealed during gastric surgery. *Surgical and Radiologic Anatomy: SRA* 36:173–80.

Huang A., Zhao H., Ling T., Quan Y., Zheng M., Feng B. 2014b. Oncological superiority of extralevator abdominoperineal resection over conventional abdominoperineal resection: a meta-analysis. *International Journal of Colorectal Disease* 29:321–7.

Huang C., Zheng C. (eds.) 2015a. Laparoscopic Suprapancreatic Area Lymph Node Dissection for Gastric Cancer. In: *Laparoscopic Gastrectomy for Gastric Cancer: Surgical Technique and Lymphadenectomy*. Springer Science+Business Media Dordrecht and People's Medical Publishing House, 97–203.

Huang C., Zheng C. (eds.) 2015b. Summary of Anatomy and Physiology of Perigastric Lymphatic System. In: *Laparoscopic Gastrectomy for Gastric Cancer: 1 Surgical Technique and Lymphadenectomy*. Springer Science+Business Media Dordrecht and People's Medical Publishing House, 1–6.

Hur M-S., Kim H-J., Lee K-S. 2015. Termination of the ligamentum venosum and the topographic relationship between the left portal vein, left hepatic artery, and ligamentum venosum in the fissures for the ligamentum teres and ligamentum venosum. *Surgical and Radiologic Anatomy: SRA* 37:449–55.

Inoue Y., Saiura A., Yoshioka R., Ono Y., Takahashi M., Arita J., Takahashi Y., Koga R. 2015. Pancreatoduodenectomy With Systematic Mesopancreas Dissection Using a Supracolic Anterior Artery-First Approach. *Annals of Surgery.*

Jamieson NB., Foulis AK., Oien KA., Going JJ., Glen P., Dickson EJ., et a. l. 2010. Positive mobilization margins alone do not influence survival following pancreatico-duodenectomy for pancreatic ductal adenocarcinoma. *Annals of Surgery* 251:1003–1010.

Jang JY., Kang MJ., Heo JS., Choi SH., Choi DW., Park SJ., Han SS., Yoon DS., Yu HC., Kang KJ., Kim SG., Kim SW. 2014. A prospective randomized controlled study comparing outcomes of standard resection and extended resection, including dissection of the nerve plexus and various lymph nodes, in patients with pancreatic head cancer. *Ann Surg.* 259:656–664.

Japan Esophageal Society. 2009. Japanese Classification of Esophageal Cancer, tenth edition: part I. *Esophagus* 6:71–94.

Japan Pancreas Society. 2003. *The English Edition of the General Rules for the Study of Pancreatic Cancer by the Japan Pancreas Society.* Tokyo: Kanehara.

Japanese Gastric Cancer Association. 2011. Japanese gastric cancer treatment guidelines 2010 (ver. 3). *Gastric cancer: official journal of the International Gastric Cancer Association and the Japanese Gastric Cancer Association* 14:113–23.

John BJ., Naik P., Ironside A., Davidson BR., Fusai G., Gillmore R., et a. l. 2013. Redefining the R1 resection for pancreatic ductal adenocarcinoma: tumour lymph nodal burden and lymph node ratio are the only prognostic factors associated with survival. *HPB: The Official Journal of the International Hepato Pancreato Biliary Association* 15:674–680.

Jones R., Poston G. 2011. Surgical anatomy of the liver and bile ducts. In: Poston G, D'Angelica M, Adam R eds. *Surgical Management of Hepatobiliary and Pancreatic Disorders.* Informa Healthcare USA, Inc., 1–16.

Kawai M., Tani M., Ina S., Hirono S., Nishioka R., Miyazawa M., et a. l. 2008. CLIP method (preoperative CT image-assessed ligation of inferior pancreaticoduodenal artery) reduces intraoperative bleeding during pancreaticoduodenectomy. *World Journal of Surgery* 32:82–87.

Kawasaki K., Kanaji S., Kobayashi I., Fujita T., Kominami H., Ueno K., Tsutida S., Ohno M., Ohsawa M., Fujino Y., Tominaga M., Nakamura T. 2010. Multidetector computed tomography for preoperative identification of left gastric vein location in patients with gastric cancer. *Gastric Cancer: Official Journal of the International Gastric Cancer Association and the Japanese Gastric Cancer Association* 13:25–9.

Kim MS., Chang X., LeBron C., Nagpal JK., Lee J., Huang Y., Yamashita K., Trink B., Ratovitski EA., Sidransky D. 2010. Neurofilament heavy polypeptide regulates the Akt-beta-catenin pathway in human esophageal squamous cell carcinoma. *PloS one* 5:e9003.

Kim DH., Choi MG., Noh JH., Sohn TS., Bae JM., Kim S. 2015. Clinical significance of skip lymph node metastasis in gastric cancer patients. *European Journal of Surgical Oncology: The Journal of the European Society of Surgical Oncology and the British Association of Surgical Oncology* 41:339–45.

Klein M., Fischer A., Rosenberg J., Gögenur I. 2015. ExtraLevatory AbdominoPerineal Excision (ELAPE) Does Not Result in Reduced Rate of Tumor Perforation or Rate of Positive Circumferential Resection Margin. *Annals of Surgery* 261:933–938.

Kondo S. 2010. Japanese Pancreas Society Staging Systems for Pancreatic Cancer. In: Neoptolemos JP, Urrutia R, Abbruzzese JL, Buchler M eds. *Pancreatic Cancer.* Springer Science+Business Media, 1036–1050.

Konstantinidis IT., Warshaw AL., Allen JN., Blaszkowsky LS., Castillo CF., Deshpande V., *et al.* 2013. Pancreatic ductal adenocarcinoma: is there a survival difference for R1 resections *versus* locally advanced unresectable tumors? What is a "true" R0 resection? *Annals of Surgery* 257:731–736.

Kooby D., Loukas M., Skandalakis L., McClusky D., Mirilas P. 2011. Surgical Anatomy of the Pancreas. In: Fishcer J ed. *Mastery of Surgery.* Wolters Kluwer Lippincott Williams and Wilkins, 1375–1392.

Krishna A., Rickard MJFX., Keshava A., Dent OF., Chapuis PH. 2013. A comparison of published rates of resection margin involvement and intra-operative perforation between standard and "cylindrical" abdominoperineal excision for low rectal cancer. *Colorectal Disease: The Official Journal of the Association of Coloproctology of Great Britain and Ireland* 15:57–65.

Lam T., Usatoff V., Chan STF. 2014. Are we getting the critical view? A prospective study of photographic documentation during laparoscopic cholecystectomy. *HPB: The Official Journal of the International Hepato Pancreato Biliary Association* 16:859–63.

Lambrecht NWG. 2011. Ménétrier's disease of the stomach: a clinical challenge. *Current Gastro-Enterology Reports* 13:513–7.

Law S. 2011. Esophagogastrectomy for Carcinoma of the Esophagus. In: Fischer J, Jones D, Pomposelli F, Upchurch Jr G eds. *Mastery of Surgery.* Wolters Kluwer Lippincott Williams and Wilkins, 886–903.

Law WL., Chu KW. 2004. Abdominoperineal resection is associated with poor oncological outcome. *The British Journal of Surgery* 91:1493–9.

Lerut T., Coosemans W., Decaluwe H., Decker G., De Leyn P., Nafteux P., Raemdonck and D Van. 2011. The Anatomy of the Esophagus. In: Fischer J, Jones D, Pomposelli F, Upchurch Jr G eds. *Mastery of Surgery.* Wolters Kluwer Lippincott Williams and Wilkins, 792–809.

Lim LG., Ho KY., So JB., Khor CJ., Lim LL., Teoh PL., Yeoh KG. 2015. Diagnosis and treatment of Helicobacter pylori for peptic ulcer bleeding in clinical practice - factors associated with non-diagnosis and non-treatment, and diagnostic yield in various settings. *The Turkish Journal of Gastroenterology* 25:157–161.

Lin PH., Chaikof EL. 2000. Embryology, anatomy, and surgical exposure of the great abdominal vessels. *The Surgical Clinics of North America* 80:417–33, xiv.

Lin JX HC. 2013. Classification of Anatomic Variations in the Left Gastric Vein during Laparoscopic Gastrectomy. *Anatomy and Physiology* 03.

Lindner HH., Kemprud E. 1971. A clinicoanatomical study of the arcuate ligament of the diaphragm. *Archives of Surgery (Chicago, Ill.: 1960)* 103:600–5.

Liu DL., Xia S., Xu W., Ye Q., Gao Y., Qian J. 1996. Anatomy of vasculature of 850 spleen specimens and its application in partial splenectomy. *Surgery* 119:27–33.

Liu P., Bao H., Zhang X., Zhang J., Ma L., Wang Y., Li C., Wang Z., Gong P. 2015. Better operative outcomes achieved with the prone jackknife vs. lithotomy position during abdominoperineal resection in patients with low rectal cancer. *World Journal of Surgical Oncology* 13:39.

Lundell L., Vieth M., Gibson F. 2015. Systematic review: the effects of long-term proton pump inhibitor use on serum gastrin levels and gastric histology. *Alimentary ....*

Maksymov V., Hogan M., Khalifa MA. 2013. An anatomical-based mapping analysis of the pancreaticoduodenectomy retroperitoneal margin highlights the urgent need for standardized assessment. *HPB: The Official Journal of the International Hepato Pancreato Biliary Association* 15:218–223.

Mandal AK., Lee H., Salem F. 1988. Review of primary tumors of the diaphragm. *Journal of the National Medical Association* 80:214–7.

Miles WE. A method of performing abdomino-perineal excision for carcinoma of the rectum and of the terminal portion of the pelvic colon (1908). *CA: A Cancer Journal for Clinicians* 21:361–4.

Mills S. 2006. *Histology for pathologists.*

Mise Y., Satou S., Shindoh J., Conrad C., Aoki T., Hasegawa K., Sugawara Y., Kokudo N. 2014. Three-dimensional volumetry in 107 normal livers reveals clinically relevant inter-segment variation in size. *HPB: The Official Journal of the International Hepato Pancreato Biliary Association* 16:439–47.

Miyaki A., Imamura K., Kobayashi R., Takami M., Matsumoto J., Takada Y. 2012. Preoperative assessment of perigastric vascular anatomy by multidetector computed tomography angiogram for laparoscopy-assisted gastrectomy. *Langenbeck's Archives of Surgery / Deutsche Gesellschaft für Chirurgie* 397:945–50.

Miyaki T., Yamada M., Kumaki K. 1987. Aberrant course of the left gastric vein in the human. Possibility of a persistent left portal vein. *Acta anatomica* 130:275–9.

Miyazawa M., Kawai M., Hirono S., Okada K., Shimizu A., Kitahata Y., Yamaue H. 2015. Preoperative evaluation of the confluent drainage veins to the gastrocolic trunk of Henle: understanding the surgical vascular anatomy during pancreaticoduodenectomy. *Journal of Hepato-Biliary-Pancreatic Sciences* 22:386–91.

Moore K., Persaud T. 2008. *The Developing Human: Clinically Oriented Embriology*. Saunders Elsevier.

Mouly C., Fuks D., Browet F., Mauvais F., Potier A., Yzet T., Quentin Q., Regimbeau J-M. 2013. Feasibility of the Glissonian approach during right hepatectomy. *HPB: The Official Journal of the International Hepato Pancreato Biliary Association* 15:638–45.

Nagakawa T., Mori K., Nakano T., Kadoya M., Kobayashi H., Akiyama T., Kayahara M., Ohta T., Ueno K., Higashino Y., Konishi I., Miyazaki I. 1993. Perineural invasion of carcinoma of the pancreas and biliary tract. *British Journal of Surgery* 80:619–621.

Nagtegaal ID., van de Velde CJH., Marijnen CAM., van Krieken JHJM., Quirke P. 2005. Low rectal cancer: a call for a change of approach in abdominoperineal resection. *Journal of Clinical Oncology: Official Journal of the American Society of Clinical Oncology* 23:9257–64.

Nair V., Fischer S., Adeyi O. 2010. Non–Viral-Related Pathologic Findings in Liver Needle Biopsy Specimens From Patients With Chronic Viral Hepatitis. *American Journal of Clinical…*.

Nakamura M., Nakashima H., Tsutsumi K., Matsumoto H., Muta Y., Ueno D., et al. 2013. First jejunal vein oriented mesenteric excision for pancreatoduodenectomy. *Journal of Gastro-Enterology* 48:989–995.

Nakao A., Harada A., Nonami T., Kaneko T., Murakami H., Inoue S., Takeuchi Y., Takagi H. 1995. Lymph node metastases in carcinoma of the head of the pancreas region. *The British Journal of Surgery* 82:399–402.

De Nardi P., Summo V., Vignali A., Capretti G. 2015. Standard Versus Extralevator Abdomino-perineal Low Rectal Cancer Excision Outcomes: A Systematic Review and Meta-analysis. *Annals of Surgical Oncology*.

Natsume T., Shuto K., Kohno T., Ohira G., Tohma T., Sato A., Saito H., Ohta T., Kawahira H., Akai T., Nabeya Y., Hayashi H., Matsubara H. 2010. Anatomic Variations of the Celiac Trunk and the Left Gastric Vein Assessing by Dual-Phase CT Angiography for Safety Laparoscopic Gastrectomy. *Journal of Surgical Research* 158:387–388.

NCCN Clinical Practice Guidelines in Oncology. 2015.Pancreatic Adenocarcinoma. *Available at http://www.nccn.org/professionals/physician_gls/pdf/pancreatic.pdf* (accessed July 14, 2015).

Negoi I., Draghia F., Draghia A., Negoi R. 2010. *Anatomy of the Digestive Tract for Students*. Carol Davila University Press.

Negoi R. 2014. Celulele germinale primordiale – implicaşii clinice. In: Filipoiu F ed. *Lucrări practice embriologie an I*. Editura Universitara Carol Davila Bucuresti, 75–85.

Negoi I., Paun S., Hostiuc S., Negoi R., Beuran M. 2015a. *Laparoscopic* versus *Open Complete Mesocolic Excision with Central Vascular Ligation for Colon Cancer – A Systematic Review and Meta-Analysis*.

Negoi I., Paun S., Hostiuc S., Negoi R., Beuran M. 2015b. *Extralevator* versus *Conventional Abdominoperineal Resection for Rectal Cancer – A Systematic Review and Meta-Analysis*. The American Journal of Surgery 2016 (in press).

Negoi I., Constantinescu N. 2015. Surigcal Anatomy of Rectum. In: *Surgical and Operative Anatomy*. Editura Academiei Oamenilor de Ştiinţă din România.

Nelson H., Petrelli N., Carlin A., Couture J., Fleshman J., Guillem J., Miedema B., Ota D., Sargent D. 2001. Guidelines 2000 for colon and rectal cancer surgery. *Journal of the National Cancer Institute* 93:583–96.

Nivatvongs S., Gordon P. 2007. Surgical Anatomy. In: Nivatvongs S, Gordon P eds. *Principles and Practice of Surgery for the Colon, Rectum, and Anus*. Informa Healthcare USA, Inc.

Noto M., Miwa K., Kitagawa H., Kayahara M., Takamura H., Shimizu K., et al. 2005. Pancreas head carcinoma: frequency of invasion to soft tissue adherent to the superior mesenteric artery. *The American Journal of Surgical Pathology* 29:1056–1061.

Oh SJ., Hyung WJ., Li C., Song J., Kang W., Rha SY., Chung HC., Choi SH., Noh SH. 2009. The effect of spleen-preserving lymphadenectomy on surgical outcomes of locally advanced proximal gastric cancer. *Journal of Surgical Oncology* 99:275–80.

Ohkubo M. 2000. Aberrant left gastric vein directly draining into the liver. *Clinical Anatomy (New York, N.Y.)* 13:134–7.

Ortiz H., Ciga MA., Armendariz P., Kreisler E., Codina-Cazador A., Gomez-Barbadillo J., Garcia-Granero E., Roig J V., Biondo S. 2014. Multicentre propensity score-matched analysis of conventional versus extended abdominoperineal excision for low rectal cancer. *British Journal of Surgery* 101:874–882.

Pallisera A., Morales R., Ramia JM. 2014. Tricks and tips in pancreatoduodenectomy. *World Journal of Gastrointestinal Oncology* 6:344–350.

Peng S. 2010. Anatomy. In: *Hepatic Caudate Lobe Resection*. Springer, 1–15.

Peparini N., Chirletti P. 2012. Clearance of the retropancreatic margin in pancreatic carcinomas: total mesopancreas excision or extended lymphadenectomy? *European Journal of Surgical Oncology: The Journal of the European Society of Surgical Oncology and the British Association of Surgical Oncology* 38:1146; author reply 1147–1146; author reply 1147.

Peparini N., Chirletti P. 2013. Mesopancreas: a boundless structure, namely R1 risk in pancreaticoduodenectomy for pancreatic head carcinoma. *European Journal of surgical Oncology: The Journal of the European Society of Surgical Oncology and the British Association of Surgical Oncology* 39:1303–1308.

Poston G., Blumgart LH. 2003. Surgical anatomy of the liver and bile ducts. In: Poston G, Blumgart LH eds. *Surgical Management of Hepatobiliary and Pancreatic Disorders*. Martin Dunitz Ltd, 1–29.

Prytz M., Angenete E., Bock D., Haglind E. 2015. Extralevator Abdominoperineal Excision for Low Rectal Cancer-Extensive Surgery to be Used With Discretion Based on 3-Year Local Recurrence Results: A Registry-based, Observational National Cohort Study. *Annals of Surgery*.

Ramsay G., Parnaby C., Mackay C., Hanlon P., Ong S., Loudon M. 2013. Analysis of outcome using a levator sparing technique of abdominoperineal excision of rectum and anus. Cylindrical ELAPE is not necessary in all patients. *European Journal of Surgical Oncology: The Journal of the European Society of Surgical Oncology and the British Association of Surgical Oncology* 39:1219–24.

Rebibo L., Chivot C., Fuks D., Sabbagh C., Yzet T., Regimbeau J-M. 2012. Three-dimensional computed tomography analysis of the left gastric vein in a pancreatectomy. *HPB: The Official Journal of the International Hepato Pancreato Biliary Association* 14:414–21.

Redmond HP., Redmond JM., Rooney BP., Duignan JP., Bouchier-Hayes DJ. 1989. Surgical anatomy of the human spleen. *The British Journal of Surgery* 76:198–201.

Rocha GA., Queiroz DMM., Mendes EN., Barbosa AJA., Lima GF., Oliveira CA. 1991. Helicobacter-Pylori Acute Gastritis – Histological, Endoscopic, Clinical, and Therapeutic Features. *American Journal of Gastroenterology* 86:1592–1595.

Rosai J. 2011. *Rosai and Ackerman's Surgical Pathology*. Elsevier.

Rozen WM., Garcia-Tutor E., Alonso-Burgos A., Corlett RJ., Taylor GI., Ashton MW. 2009. The effect of anterior abdominal wall scars on the vascular anatomy of the abdominal wall: A cadaveric and clinical study with clinical implications. *Clinical Anatomy (New York, N.Y.)* 22:815–22.

Rozen WM., Ashton MW., Taylor GI. 2008. Reviewing the vascular supply of the anterior abdominal wall: redefining anatomy for increasingly refined surgery. *Clinical Anatomy (New York, N.Y.)* 21:89–98.

Rüdiger Siewert J., Feith M., Werner M., Stein HJ. 2000. Adenocarcinoma of the esophagogastric junction: results of surgical therapy based on anatomical/topographic classification in 1,002 consecutive patients. *Annals of Surgery* 232:353–61.

Sadler T. 2009. *Langman's Medical Embryology*. Wolters Kluwer Lippincott Williams and Wilkins.

Sanjay P., Takaori K., Govil S., Shrikhande S V., Windsor JA. 2012. "Artery-first" approaches to pancreatoduodenectomy. *The British Journal of Surgery* 99:1027–1035.

Sano T., Sasako M., Yamamoto S., Nashimoto A., Kurita A., Hiratsuka M., Tsujinaka T., Kinoshita T., Arai K., Yamamura Y., Okajima K. 2004. Gastric cancer surgery: morbidity and mortality results from a prospective randomized controlled trial comparing D2 and extended para-aortic lymphadenectomy – Japan Clinical Oncology Group study 9501. *Journal of Clinical Oncology: Official Journal of the American Society of Clinical Oncology* 22:2767–73.

Sareli M., Chanukvadze I., Valeanu A., Zippel DB., Shapiro R., Papa MZ. 2009. The posterior intrahepatic approach to the left portal pedicle using the ligamentum venosum: anatomical basis. *Surgical and Radiologic Anatomy: SRA* 31:809–13.

Sasako M., Sano T., Yamamoto S., Kurokawa Y., Nashimoto A., Kurita A., Hiratsuka M., Tsujinaka T., Kinoshita T., Arai K., Yamamura Y., Okajima K. 2008. D2 lymphadenectomy alone or with para-aortic nodal dissection for gastric cancer. *The New England Journal of Medicine* 359:453–62.

Schaffner F., Popper H. 1985. Classification and mechanism of cholestasis. *Wright R, Albert KGMM, Karran S, Millvard-Sadler GDT.....*

Schwarz RE. 2002. Spleen-preserving splenic hilar lymphadenectomy at the time of gastrectomy for cancer: technical feasibility and early results. *Journal of Surgical Oncology* 79:73–6.

Selmi C., Bowlus C., Gershwin M., Coppel R. 2011. Primary biliary cirrhosis. *The Lancet*.

Sen S., Dişcigil B., Badak I., Gürcün U. 2007. Lipoma of the diaphragm: a rare presentation. *The Annals of Thoracic Surgery* 83:2203–5.

Shimizu J., Hashimoto T., Imai T., Kawahara E. 1996. Primary lipoma of the diaphragm. *Respiration; International Review of Thoracic Diseases* 63:397–9.

Shoup S., Smith J. 2011. Anatomy of the pancreas. In: Poston G, D'Angelica M, Adam R eds. *Surgical Management of Hepatobiliary and Pancreatic Disorders*. Informa Healthcare USA, Inc., 17–24.

Shukla PJ., Barreto SG., Kulkarni A., Nagarajan G., Fingerhut A. 2010. Vascular anomalies encountered during pancreatoduodenectomy: do they influence outcomes? *Annals of Surgical Oncology* 17:186–193.

Skandalakis J., Colburn G., Weidman T., Foster Jr R., Kingsworth A., Skandalakis L., Skandalakis P., Mirilas P. 2004. *Skandalakis' Surgical Anatomy: The Embryologic and Anatomic Basis of Modern Surgery*. Paschalidis Medical Publications, Ltd.

Songun I., Putter H., Kranenbarg EM-K., Sasako M., van de Velde CJH. 2010. Surgical treatment of gastric cancer: 15-year follow-up results of the randomised nationwide Dutch D1D2 trial. *The Lancet. Oncology* 11:439–49.

Spitz L., Kiely E., Brereton RJ. 1987. Esophageal atresia: five year experience with 148 cases. *Journal of Pediatric Surgery* 22:103–8.

Stange D., Weitz J. 2015. Methods of Reconstruction – BI, BII, Roux-en-Y, Jejunal Interposition, Proximal Gastrectomy and Pouch Reconstruction. In: Strong V ed. *Gastric Cancer*. Springer International Publishing Switzerland, 175–183.

Stelzner F. 2007. Mesorectum, is it an appropriate term? by A. Tufano *et al. International Journal of Colorectal Disease* 22:1129–30.

Strasberg S., Belghiti J., Clavien P., Gadzijev E., Garden J., Lau W., Makuuchi M., Strong R. 2000. The Brisbane 2000 Terminology of Liver Anatomy and Resections. *HPB (Oxford)* 2:333–339.

Strasberg S. 2010. Hepatic Anatomy and Terminology. In: Clavien P ed. *Malignant Liver Tumors: Current and Emerging Therapies*. Blackwell Publishing, 11–26.

Strasberg SM., Gouma DJ. 2012. "Extreme" vasculobiliary injuries: association with fundus-down cholecystectomy in severely inflamed gallbladders. *HPB: The Official Journal of the International Hepato Pancreato Biliary Association* 14:1–8.

Strasberg SM., Helton WS. 2011. An analytical review of vasculobiliary injury in laparoscopic and open cholecystectomy. *HPB: The Official Journal of the International Hepato Pancreato Biliary Association* 13:1–14.

Strasberg SM., Hertl M., Soper NJ. 1995. An analysis of the problem of biliary injury during laparoscopic cholecystectomy. *Journal of the American College of Surgeons* 180:101–25.

Strasberg SM., Phillips C. 2013. Use and dissemination of the brisbane 2000 nomenclature of liver anatomy and resections. *Annals of Surgery* 257:377–82.

Sugarbaker PH. 2015. A Patent Cranial End of the Ductus Venosus Can Result in Hemorrhage when Performing a Lesser Omentectomy-Omental Bursectomy Procedure. *Annals of Surgical Oncology*.

Takahashi T., Ueno M., Azekura K., Ohta H. 2000. Lateral node dissection and total mesorectal excision for rectal cancer. *Diseases of the Colon and Rectum* 43:S59–S68.

Takemura N., Hasegawa K., Sugawara Y., Zhang K., Aoki T., Beck Y., Makuuchi M., Kokudo N. 2010. Morphometric analysis of caudate veins for advanced liver surgery. *HPB: The Official Journal of the International Hepato Pancreato Biliary Association* 12:619–24.

Tang S., Wu R., Bhaijee F. 2014. Zollinger–Ellison Syndrome. ... *Journal and Encyclopedia of GI Endoscopy*.

Tung T. 1939. La vascularisation veineuse du foie et ses applications aux resections hepatiques. Hanoi.

Tung T. 1979. *Les Resections Majeures et Mineures du Foie*. Masson Paris.

Verbeke CS., Menon K V. 2009. Redefining resection margin status in pancreatic cancer. *HPB: The Official Journal of the International Hepato Pancreato Biliary Association* 11:282–289.

Vettoretto N., Saronni C., Harbi A., Balestra L., Taglietti L., Giovanetti M. Critical view of safety during laparoscopic cholecystectomy. *JSLS: Journal of the Society of Laparoendoscopic Surgeons / Society of Laparoendoscopic Surgeons* 15:322–5.

Watanabe T., Itabashi M., Shimada Y., Tanaka S., Ito Y., Ajioka Y., Hamaguchi T., Hyodo I., Igarashi M., Ishida H., Ishiguro M., Kanemitsu Y., Kokudo N., Muro K., Ochiai A., Oguchi M., Ohkura Y., Saito Y., Sakai Y., Ueno H., Yoshino T., Fujimori T., Koinuma N., Morita T., Nishimura G., Sakata Y., Takahashi K., Takiuchi H., Tsuruta O., Yamaguchi T., Yoshida M., Yamaguchi N., Kotake K., Sugihara K. 2012. Japanese Society for Cancer of the Colon and Rectum (JSCCR) guidelines 2010 for the treatment of colorectal cancer. *International Journal of Clinical Oncology* 17:1–29.

West NP., Hohenberger W., Weber K., Perrakis A., Finan PJ., Quirke P. 2010a. Complete mesocolic excision with central vascular ligation produces an oncologically superior specimen compared with standard surgery for carcinoma of the colon. *Journal of Clinical Oncology* 28:272–278.

West NP., Anderin C., Smith KJE., Holm T., Quirke P. 2010b. Multicentre experience with extralevator abdominoperineal excision for low rectal cancer. *The British Journal of Surgery* 97:588–99.

West NP., Kobayashi H., Takahashi K., Perrakis A., Weber K., Hohenberger W., Sugihara K., Quirke P. 2012. Understanding optimal colonic cancer surgery: Comparison of Japanese D3 resection and european complete mesocolic excision with central vascular ligation. *Journal of Clinical Oncology* 30:1763–1769.

Wexner S., Jorge J. 2005. Anatomy and Embriology of the Anus, Rectum and Colon. In: Corman M ed. *Colon and Rectal Surgery*. Lippincott Williams and Wilkins, 16.

Whitehead R., Truelove SC., Gear MW. 1972. The histological diagnosis of chronic gastritis in fibreoptic gastroscope biopsy specimens. *Journal of Clinical Pathology* 25:1–11.

Wu CW., Hsiung CA., Lo SS., Hsieh MC., Shia LT., Whang-Peng J. 2004. Randomized clinical trial of morbidity after D1 and D3 surgery for gastric cancer. *The British Journal of Surgery* 91:283–7.

Yang SH., Yin YH., Jang JY., Lee SE., Chung JW., Suh KS., et a. l. 2007. Assessment of hepatic arterial anatomy in keeping with preservation of the vasculature while performing pancreatoduodenectomy: an opinion. *World Journal of Surgery* 31:2384–2391.

Yang L., Zhao X., Li A., Sheng J. 2015. Ménétrier's disease with normal albumin level. *Endoscopy.*
Yao K. 2014. *Zoom Gastroscopy.* Tokyo: Springer Japan.
Yu H-C., Peng H., He X-S., Zhao R-S. 2014. Comparison of short- and long-term outcomes after extralevator abdominoperineal excision and standard abdominoperineal excision for rectal cancer: a systematic review and meta-analysis. *International Journal of Colorectal Disease* 29:183–91.
Zhou X., Sun T., Xie H., Zhang Y., Zeng H., Wei F. 2015. Extralevator abdominoperineal excision for low rectal cancer: a systematic review and meta-analysis of the short-term outcome. *Colorectal Disease: The Official Journal of the Association of Coloproctology of Great Britain and Ireland* 17:474–81.